KT-119-377

| | |
|---|---|
| Pre-travel health assessment | 5 |
| Geographical distribution of health hazards | 9 |
| Individuals with special considerations | 14 |
| Motion sickness and jet lag | 24 |
| Vaccines | 28 |
| Malaria | 41 |
| Other mosquito-transmitted diseases | 55 |
| Food- and water-borne illnesses | 64 |
| Other parasitic diseases | 83 |
| Diseases transmitted by ticks, lice, mites and fleas | 92 |
| Miscellaneous infectious diseases | 98 |
| Environmental and climatic factors | 111 |
| Returned travellers | 123 |
| Appendices | 130 |
| Key references | 144 |
| Index | 149 |

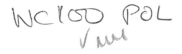

# FAST FACTS

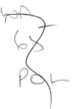

# Travel Medicine

Indispensab˙
Guides to
Clinical
Practice

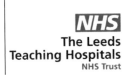

Oxford

Fast Facts – Travel Medicine
First published March 2001

CHAPTER 1
# Pre-travel health assessment

Over recent decades, the number of people travelling internationally has grown dramatically. There has also been an increase in the speed of global travel and the accessibility of remote areas to tourists. These factors all serve to expose a large number of people to health hazards they might not otherwise encounter.

Giving advice to travellers prior to departure is largely an exercise in risk assessment. Not only is it necessary to know the potential health hazards of the chosen destination, it is important to consider the type of activities that will be undertaken while on holiday, the type of accommodation, the duration of travel and the regional seasonal differences in the distribution of certain diseases within a country. For example, the health risks for a person making a 4-day business trip to Bangkok are likely to be very different from a 20-year-old backpacker trekking in northern Thailand. The latter will be at greater risk for several infectious diseases, and will consequently receive different recommendations about vaccinations and antimalarial chemoprophylaxis. Both need similar advice, however, about the prevention of travellers' diarrhoea.

Important considerations for the physician undertaking pre-travel health assessments include:
- allowing sufficient time
- personalizing advice
- understanding the epidemiology of health hazards
- identifying high-risk groups
- encouraging individual responsibility
- discussing health insurance
- keeping up to date.

## Allowing sufficient time
In general, travellers should be encouraged to seek advice at least 6 weeks before departure. This will allow sufficient time for vaccines, the administration of which may need to be spaced chronologically to enable optimal immunity to develop. Travellers with chronic medical conditions or

other special considerations should seek advice as early as possible. Health professionals must provide ample time for the pre-travel consultation, and for the initial clinic visit in particular.

## Personalizing advice

Pre-travel advice needs to be tailored for the individual. Specific considerations are given in Table 1.1.

## Understanding the epidemiology of health hazards

It is essential for health professionals to be familiar with both the health hazards in specific travel destinations, particularly developing countries, and the level of risk involved (Figure 1.1). Some diseases that have traditionally attracted considerable attention, such as cholera, may be encountered only rarely by travellers. For many years, a cholera vaccine with poor protective efficacy was administered widely to travellers, though in reality there was only a very small chance of exposure. Conversely, motor-vehicle accidents are a relatively common cause of injury and the single most common cause of death among travellers, yet are rarely discussed. Much of the travel medicine literature has focused on the developing world, and the fact that

---

TABLE 1.1

**Special considerations during the pre-travel assessment**

- Traveller's age
- Previous vaccination history
- Medical history, including
  - drug allergies
  - current medications
  - past history of hepatitis
- Pregnancy
- Type of activities likely to be undertaken while travelling
- Type of travel
  - type of accommodation
  - modes of transportation

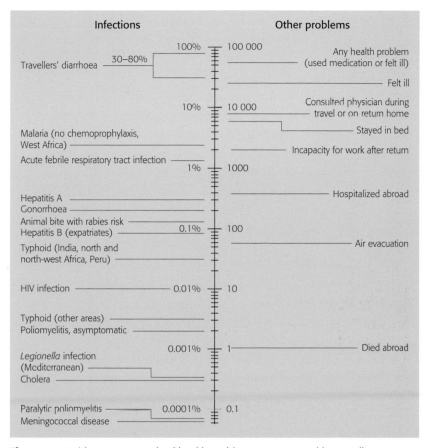

**Figure 1.1** Incidence per month of health problems encountered by travellers to developing countries. Adapted from International Travel and Health, WHO, 1998.

travel to industrialized countries is not without risk is often overlooked. When appropriate, provide the traveller with written information.

## Identifying high-risk groups

Individuals who may be at increased risk while travelling need to seek pre-travel advice early, and include:

- those with chronic diseases, including the immunocompromised, and/or complex medical problems
- pregnant women
- children

7

- long-term travellers
- those at risk for sexually transmissible diseases.

## Encouraging individual responsibility

Many health problems encountered during travel are preventable, so travellers must be encouraged to behave safely to prevent illness and injury, and to respond appropriately should either occur. Education is the cornerstone, and travellers should be provided with information about risks and the means to minimize them. Important areas to discuss are:

- safe eating and drinking to prevent food-borne illness
- injury prevention
- personal protection against biting arthropods
- safe sex
- risks of blood-borne infections.

## Discussing health insurance

Although a much neglected area, travellers should ensure that they have adequate health insurance cover, not only to meet medical care expenses, but to provide access to emergency medical assistance. Travellers to remote areas should check whether their insurance covers emergency evacuation (e.g. by helicopter).

## Keeping up to date

Disease epidemiology, travel regulations, vaccine availability and many other issues relevant to travellers change continually. Health professionals who regularly give advice to travellers must endeavour to keep up to date with this information. The resources in Appendix A are useful in this regard.

CHAPTER 2
# Geographical distribution of health hazards

The degree of risk to which a traveller will be exposed for a particular condition varies considerably from region to region; in reality, it is very difficult, if not impossible, to define. The quality of disease epidemiological data is also variable. Consequently, most information here should serve only as a guideline to be supplemented with more specific local information. Appendix B provides country-specific data on disease risks and vaccination recommendations.

## Africa

**North Africa** encompasses Morocco, Algeria, Tunisia, Libya and Egypt. Malaria is limited to specific foci within the region and is susceptible to chloroquine. Diarrhoeal diseases and typhoid are common, and hepatitis A (and probably E) is endemic. Schistosomiasis occurs in foci, but is particularly common in the Nile River Valley. Other diseases affecting travellers less commonly include leishmaniasis, brucellosis, hydatid disease, typhus, rabies, relapsing fever, Rift Valley fever and West Nile fever.

**Sub-Saharan Africa** comprises the bulk of the African continent, and includes countries from the Sahara desert in the north to Angola, Zambia and Mozambique in the south. Specific health risks vary considerably across the region. Malaria is endemic throughout the region, except above 2500 m and in certain urban areas. Other important arthropod-borne diseases include yellow fever, trypanosomiasis, leishmaniasis, onchocerciasis (river blindness) and other viral haemorrhagic fevers. Diarrhoeal diseases, typhoid, intestinal helminthic infections and hydatids are common, and cases of poliomyelitis continue to be reported. Schistosomiasis is present throughout the region and is a particular risk for travellers who swim in lakes and rivers. Hepatitis A, B, C and E are endemic. Meningococcal meningitis epidemics occur, particularly within the 'meningitis belt' during the dry season. HIV is common in this region. Other notable hazards include snakes and rabies. Altitude illness is possible in several areas, and is particularly common among travellers climbing Kilimanjaro.

**Southern Africa** includes Namibia, Botswana, Zimbabwe, South Africa, Lesotho and Swaziland. Malaria is present in certain areas, particularly in the north. HIV infection is common throughout Southern Africa. Trypanosomiasis occurs in Botswana and Namibia. Other arthropod-borne diseases are generally less common than in sub-Saharan Africa. Diarrhoeal diseases, typhoid, hepatitis A and B, and schistosomiasis are endemic. Poliomyelitis is now very uncommon.

## The Americas
**North America.** Health risks in Canada and the USA are unlikely to be greater than in the traveller's home country. Hazards in certain areas include Lyme disease, rabies, plague, Rocky Mountain spotted fever, erhlichiosis, tularaemia, viral encephalitides, hantavirus infection, histoplasmosis, blastomycosis, coccidioidomycosis, and fish and shellfish poisoning. Extremes of temperature can be problematic at certain times of the year. The risk of food-borne illness is generally low.

**Central America** includes the mainland countries from Mexico in the north to Panama in the south. Malaria occurs in foci throughout the region, and is chloroquine susceptible. Diarrhoeal diseases, typhoid and hepatitis A are common, while leishmaniasis, Chagas' disease, rabies and dengue have been reported in all countries. Histoplasmosis and brucellosis are present in some areas.

**The Caribbean** encompasses the island nations of the Caribbean Sea and Bermuda. In many tourist resorts, health risks differ little from the travellers' home countries. However, there is generally a higher risk of diarrhoeal diseases and hepatitis A. Malaria occurs only in Haiti and the Dominican Republic. Schistosomiasis is endemic in the Dominican Republic, Guadeloupe, Martinique, Puerto Rico and St Lucia. Dengue is reported occasionally, and rabies exists on some islands. In the sea, jellyfish and sea-urchins are hazardous.

**Tropical South America** includes Ecuador, Columbia, Venezuela, Guyana, Suriname, French Guiana, Peru, Brazil, Bolivia and Paraguay. Malaria occurs in the low-altitude areas of all countries, particularly in the Amazon

Basin and chloroquine-resistant *Plasmodium falciparum* malaria is common. Chagas' disease, leishmaniasis (cutaneous, mucocutaneous and visceral) and onchocerciasis are endemic in some areas. Yellow fever is found in forested areas to the east of the Andes. Diarrhoeal diseases and hepatitis A are common. Schistosomiasis occurs in parts of Brazil, Venezuela and Suriname. Other diseases occasionally reported include dengue, rabies, Oroya fever, louse-borne typhus and viral encephalitides. Travellers to high-altitude areas in the Andes are at risk for altitude illness.

**Temperate South America** includes Chile, Uruguay, Argentina and the Falkland Islands. Malaria is occasionally found in north-west Argentina, but generally this area is malaria-free. Diarrhoeal diseases and hepatitis A are relatively common. Chagas' disease and cutaneous leishmaniasis are present in the north of this region, but the risk is lower than in tropical South America. Anthrax is still reported from some areas. Travellers to high-altitude areas in the Andes are at risk for altitude illness.

## Asia
**East Asia** includes China, Mongolia, North Korea, South Korea, Japan and Taiwan. Malaria is endemic in focal areas of southern China. There have also been recent reports of malaria from some areas on the Korean peninsula, but travellers are uncommon in these areas. Diarrhoeal diseases and hepatitis are common, though the risk is low in Japan, South Korea and Hong Kong. Liver, lung and intestinal fluke infections are common in places, particularly in parts of China. Schistosomiasis is endemic in the Yangtze River basin in China. Dengue, Japanese encephalitis, Korean haemorrhagic fever and scrub typhus occur in some areas, and plague is still reported from China and Mongolia.

**South-East Asia** encompasses Myanmar, Laos, Vietnam, Thailand, Cambodia, Malaysia, Singapore, Philippines, Brunei and Indonesia. Malaria is present in all countries except Singapore and Brunei. Mefloquine-resistant *P. falciparum* malaria occurs along the Thai–Myanmar and Thai–Cambodian borders. Diarrhoeal diseases and hepatitis A are common, though the risk is low in Singapore. Liver, lung and intestinal fluke infections are common in some areas, particularly on the Indo-China peninsula.

Japanese encephalitis, dengue and typhus are endemic in certain areas. Schistosomiasis occurs in foci in the southern Philippines, Sulawesi, the Mekong River delta and southern Vietnam. Melioidosis has been reported throughout the region.

**Indian subcontinent** includes India, Pakistan, Nepal, Bangladesh and Bhutan, plus the surrounding countries of Sri Lanka, the Maldives, Afghanistan and the former soviet central Asian republics (Kazakhstan, Kyrgyzstan, Tajikistan, Turkmenistan and Uzbekistan). Malaria is endemic in many low-altitude areas. Diarrhoeal diseases, typhoid, and hepatitis A and E are very common. Japanese encephalitis is common in the Indian subcontinent and Sri Lanka. Other, usually focal, diseases include leishmaniasis, typhus, dengue and plague. Hepatitis B is endemic, and rabies is present in all countries. Outbreaks of meningococcal meningitis have occurred in Nepal and the mountains of northern India. Altitude illness is common among travellers to high-altitude destinations.

**The Middle East** extends from Turkey in the north-west to Iran in the east and the Arabian peninsula in the south. Foci of malaria exist throughout the region, though the risk is generally low. Diarrhoeal diseases and hepatitis A are common. Hepatitis B is endemic and cutaneous leishmaniasis is present throughout the region. Heat-related disorders are a particular hazard.

## Europe
**Eastern Europe** includes Russia, the former soviet European republics (Estonia, Latvia, Lithuania, Belarus, Ukraine and Moldova), Slovenia, Croatia, Bosnia, Herzegovina, Yugoslavia, Hungary, Czech Republic, Slovakia and Poland. The risk of diarrhoeal diseases varies from moderate to low. Fish tapeworm (diphyllobothriasis) may be present in freshwater fish around the Baltic Sea. Tick-borne encephalitis and Lyme disease are present in many forested areas, and rabies is endemic in certain rural areas. Recent epidemics of diphtheria have occurred in Russia, Belarus and Ukraine.

**Western Europe** includes Scandinavia, the British Isles, and mainland Europe from Germany, Austria and Greece in the east to Portugal and Spain in the west. The risk of diarrhoeal diseases is generally low. Tick-borne encephalitis and Lyme disease occur in forested regions, particularly in the east and south. Leishmaniasis, and sporadic cases of typhus and West Nile fever occur along the Mediterranean littoral.

## Australasia

**Australia and New Zealand.** The risk of diarrhoeal diseases is low. Sporadic or regular outbreaks of several arthropod-borne viral infections in Australia include dengue, Ross River fever, Murray Valley encephalitis and Japanese encephalitis. Although both countries are rabies-free, a rabies-like lyssavirus has recently been identified in Australian fruitbats and has been implicated in human disease. Sea hazards include corals and jellyfish.

**Melanesia, Micronesia and Polynesia** cover a large number of island states in the Pacific Ocean not covered elsewhere. Malaria is endemic in Papua New Guinea, Vanuatu and the Solomon Islands; chloroquine resistance is high. The risk for diarrhoeal diseases and hepatitis A is generally moderate. Fish and shellfish poisoning is common in some areas, and angiostrongyliasis has been reported in several south Pacific islands. Dengue epidemics have occurred on most islands.

## Antarctica

The main health hazards for travellers to Antarctica are exposure to extreme cold, and remoteness should medical assistance be required. Most of the continent is above 2500 m elevation, so altitude illness can also be a problem.

CHAPTER 3
# Individuals with special considerations

Several groups of travellers are at increased risk for developing health problems during travel and deserve particular attention.

## Pregnancy

Pregnancy itself is not a contraindication to travel, unless there are complications or labour is imminent. However, pregnant women and their unborn children can be at additional risk from certain infections, vaccinations and environmental factors. Moreover, there may be uncertainties about available obstetric facilities should delivery occur during travel. Generally, the middle trimester is considered to be the safest time to travel; the American College of Obstetrics and Gynecology recommend travelling between 18 and 24 weeks' gestation. At this time, the risks of spontaneous abortion and premature labour are lowest, and women are usually feeling their best.

**Air travel.** Most airlines have restrictions about when they will allow pregnant women to fly. In general, airlines will not carry women over 36 weeks' gestation, except when travel is unavoidable. There are generally no restrictions for women between 24 and 36 weeks' gestation, unless there are pregnancy complications. It is advisable to contact individual airlines prior to travel to ascertain their regulations. Many carriers request that pregnant women carry a letter from their doctor. There are no travel restrictions for women less than 28 weeks' gestation.

In addition to the risk of going into labour, pregnant women are at increased risk of deep venous thrombosis during air travel. Concerns about the risk of cosmic radiation exposure to the fetus during prolonged air travel have prompted some authorities to recommend restricting travel to less than 200 hours during pregnancy.

**Malaria** during pregnancy (particularly falciparum malaria) is associated with significant morbidity and mortality for both mother and fetus. It is therefore recommended that, if possible, pregnant women avoid travelling to malarious areas, and particularly areas with high rates of chloroquine-resistant *P. falciparum*. If such travel is necessary, the usual personal protection measures and chemoprophylaxis are recommended (see page 44).

Chloroquine, proguanil and mefloquine appear to be safe during pregnancy, including the first trimester. Some authorities, however, recommend that mefloquine be taken during the second and third trimesters only. Doxycycline is contraindicated during pregnancy. In general, chloroquine is recommended for areas with little or no chloroquine resistance, while mefloquine alone or chloroquine with proguanil is recommended for other regions. Ideally, travel to mefloquine-resistant areas should be deferred.

**Vaccination.** Although evidence is lacking, inactivated vaccines should be avoided, if possible, during the first trimester (Table 3.1). Live vaccines should be avoided during pregnancy.

**Food-borne illness** is a particular worry in pregnant women. They should be advised to drink only boiled water, avoid pre-prepared salads, and eat well-cooked meat and pasteurized dairy products to prevent travellers' diarrhoea and other food-borne illnesses such as listeriosis and toxoplasmosis.

**High altitude** during pregnancy is associated with intrauterine growth retardation and increased rates of pregnancy-induced hypertension. These complications have been noted mainly above 2700 m. The risk associated with short-term, high-altitude journeys is unclear, though some authorities recommend that travel to above 2500 m during the first trimester be avoided.

## Children

**Preparation.** Destination is the most important consideration when travelling with children. A holiday that is suitable for adults may hold little interest for children. Many travel destinations, such as remote regions and non-industrialized countries, do not provide a safe environment.

**The journey.** Travelling with children can be rewarding both for parents and children. However, the journey itself, particularly long-haul international

TABLE 3.1

## Vaccines in pregnancy

| Vaccine | Use during pregnancy |
| --- | --- |
| *Live vaccines* | |
| Measles/mumps/rubella | Contraindicated |
| Oral poliomyelitis (OPV) | Only if substantial risk of exposure exists |
| Yellow fever | Contraindicated, unless exposure to yellow fever virus is unavoidable. If required for legal purposes only, obtain a doctor's letter of exemption |
| Typhoid Ty21a | Safety data unavailable. Risk of vaccination must be weighed against risk of disease |
| *Inactivated vaccines* | |
| Inactivated poliomyelitis (IPV) | If sufficient time prior to travel, IPV should be given as an alternative to OPV. If immediate protection is required, OPV should be given |
| Hepatitis A | Safety data unavailable. Risk of vaccination must be weighed against risk of disease |
| Hepatitis B | Can be given during pregnancy |
| Japanese encephalitis | Safety data unavailable. Risk of vaccination needs to be weighed against risk of disease |
| Rabies | If substantial risk of exposure exists. Administer if indicated |
| Influenza | Administer if indicated |
| Typhoid | Safety data unavailable. Risk of vaccination needs to be weighed against risk of disease |
| Cholera | Safety data unavailable. Risk of vaccination needs to be weighed against risk of disease |
| Meningococcal | Administer if indicated |
| Pneumococcal | Administer if indicated |
| *Toxoid* | |
| Tetanus/diphtheria | Can be given during pregnancy. Administer if indicated |
| Immunoglobulins | Administer if indicated |

Adapted from Centers for Disease Control and Prevention, 1999 flights and lengthy motor-vehicle journeys, is often the most difficult part of the holiday. Advance preparation should include careful consideration of entertainment and distractions to overcome boredom. Frequent stops should be built into the itinerary where practical. Sedatives should be avoided, as they are not indicated to treat normal childhood behaviour, but should be available to treat a disturbed, unsettled child. Chloral hydrate or promethazine are the usual choices; both can depress respiration and should be used during infancy only on medical advice.

*Pressure changes* in an aircraft can be a particular problem for a child who is unable to equalize pressure in the middle ear effectively. Children with concurrent upper respiratory tract infection or allergic rhinitis are particularly affected. Ideally travel should be delayed until symptoms resolve, but this is not usually practical. Decongestants at age-appropriate doses may provide some relief.

*Motion sickness.* Cinnarizine is recommended for severe cases, but drug use should be avoided when possible. General measures to avoid travel sickness are considered in Chapter 4.

**Malaria.** Prophylaxis is essential for children travelling to malarious regions (see Chapter 6). It is difficult to ensure that young children follow all preventive measures so extra care is required. Insect repellent should be applied to exposed areas at dawn and dusk. Always check the manufacturers' recommendations before using these agents on children.

**Food-borne illness.** Children are more susceptible to gastroenteritis than adults and are more likely to develop subsequent complications. Special care should be taken to avoid exposing children to contaminated food and water (see Chapter 8). Diarrhoea and vomiting in children should be managed aggressively with oral rehydration and antibiotics. Antimotility drugs, such as loperamide, should be avoided.

**Vaccinations.** Most vaccines can be used at all ages, but there are some exceptions and cautions (Table 3.2) (see Chapter 5).

**Altitude** sickness is probably as common in children as it is in adults. However, young children, particularly those under 5 years of age, are less

TABLE 3.2

**Vaccines not recommended at certain ages**

| Vaccine | Lower age limit |
| --- | --- |
| Hepatitis A | 2 years |
| Influenza | 6 months |
| Japanese encephalitis | 1 year |
| Lyme disease | 15 years |
| Measles | 6 months |
| Measles, mumps and rubella | 12 months |
| Meningococcal ACYW135 | 2 years |
| Pneumococcal polysaccharide | 2 years |
| Typhoid Vi | 2 years |
| Typhoid Ty21A | 6 years |
| Varicella | 12 months |
| Yellow fever | 9 months |

likely to report the symptoms of altitude illness, leading to delays in diagnosis and initiating descent. Older children are better able to report symptoms of altitude-related illness, making higher ascent possible, if undertaken cautiously with sufficient time for acclimatization. There is often no justification for taking young children to high mountain sites. There is also some evidence that infants may be at increased risk of sudden infant death syndrome at altitude.

**Environment and climate.** Children are more prone to solar and cold injury than adults. Adequate protection against sunburn with clothing, hats, sunblock cream and sunglasses is essential. In many countries, sunblock preparations particularly suitable for children are available. Children are also susceptible to heat-related illness and appropriate clothing for hot climates is necessary, as well as adequate hydration.

Their high surface area to volume ratio and thin layer of subcutaneous tissue make children susceptible to hypothermia. Children must be adequately clothed for insulation, wind- and waterproofing, and cold climates.

## Cardiovascular disease

People with well-controlled cardiovascular disease who are asymptomatic while performing everyday activities generally have no problems travelling, or even exercising at altitudes up to 3000 m. The following conditions, however, are contraindications to air travel:

- acute myocardial infarction within 4 weeks
- angina brought on by normal everyday activities
- uncontrolled congestive heart failure, hypertension or arrhythmias
- cerebrovascular accident within 3 weeks.

Supplementary oxygen may be available on some airlines. Sufficient medication should always be carried in hand luggage, together with a doctor's letter including details of the condition and treatment.

## Chronic lung disease

Healthy passengers tolerate the moderate reduction in oxygen tension associated with air travel. However, this may result in significant hypoxaemia in travellers with chronic lung disease. Air travel should not be undertaken if the traveller has:

- any condition resulting in shortness of breath at rest
- requirement for oxygen to perform normal everyday activities
- active bronchospasm
- pneumothorax within 10 days
- serious active respiratory infections, including active pulmonary tuberculosis
- thoracic surgery within 3 weeks
- otitis media or recent middle ear surgery – patients should check with their surgeon.

People with chronic lung disease should consult their doctor prior to travel to assess risks and to allow time for stabilization. The availability of supplementary oxygen may need to be discussed with the airline. Sufficient medication should always be carried in hand luggage, together with a doctor's letter containing details of the condition and treatment.

## Diabetes

Diabetic travellers are exposed to several factors that may affect blood glucose control, including time-zone and dietary changes, intercurrent illness and varying amounts of exercise. Pre-travel assessment and education is essential, and blood glucose control should be optimal at the time of departure. Sufficient equipment and medication should be taken to cover the entire trip and longer. Alternatively, medication may be purchased in the destination country, but availability should be confirmed prior to departure. Ideally, insulin should be kept refrigerated, though it will keep for at least 1 month unrefrigerated if protected from freezing and temperatures above 30°C. A few blood glucose meters may be inconsistent and inaccurate in some environmental conditions, such as above 2000 m.

Dose and timing of medication adjustments may be required during air travel. Travellers with type 2 diabetes taking oral hypoglycaemics can take medications as prescribed according to the local time regardless of time-zone changes. For diabetics on insulin who are travelling over fewer than five time

TABLE 3.3

**Insulin dose adjustment for time-zone travel**

**Travelling west across six or more time zones (i.e. long day)**

|  | Day of departure |
| --- | --- |
| Single-dose schedule | Usual dose |
| Two-dose schedule | Usual morning and evening doses |

**Travelling east across six or more time zones (i.e. short day)**

|  | Day of departure | First morning at destination |
| --- | --- | --- |
| Single-dose schedule | Usual dose | Two-thirds usual dose |
| Two-dose schedule | Usual morning and evening doses | Two-thirds usual morning dose |

Adapted from Benson E, Metz R, 1984–1985

zones, adhering to the usual schedule using local time is usually sufficient. Blood glucose should be measured regularly, and additional insulin may be necessary. For those travelling across six or more time zones, Table 3.3 shows the insulin adjustments required.

## HIV infection

There are several issues of particular importance in HIV-infected travellers.

- Many countries restrict entry to travellers with HIV infection; information relevant to the destination should be obtained prior to departure.
- Many infections encountered by travellers are associated with increased morbidity in HIV-infected individuals.
- Pre-travel vaccination advice is different for those with HIV infection. Live vaccines are generally contraindicated and the antibody response to any vaccination may be diminished.
- HIV-infected individuals may be taking complex medication regimens and may need to carry large drug supplies.

| Eighteen hours after morning dose | First morning at destination |
| --- | --- |
| If blood glucose is more than 13 mmol/litre, take one-third of usual dose followed by meal or snack | Usual dose |
| If blood glucose is more than 13 mmol/litre, take one-third of usual morning dose followed by meal or snack | Usual dose |

| Ten hours after morning dose | Second day at destination |
| --- | --- |
| If blood glucose is more than 13 mmol/litre, take remaining one-third of morning dose | Usual dose |
| If blood glucose is more than 13 mmol/litre, take usual evening dose plus remaining one-third of morning dose | Usual dose |

TABLE 3.4

**Vaccinations for HIV-infected travellers**

| Vaccine | Type | Recommendation |
|---|---|---|
| Bacillus Calmette-Guérin | Live | Contraindicated |
| Cholera | Inactivated | Generally not indicated |
| Hepatitis A | Inactivated | Probably safe |
| Immune globulin | Passive | Probably safe |
| Japanese encephalitis | Inactivated | Probably safe |
| Measles | Live | Contraindicated |
| Meningococcus | Inactivated | Probably safe |
| Polio | Killed | Probably safe |
| | Live oral | Contraindicated |
| Rabies (HDCV) | Inactivated | Probably safe |
| Typhoid | Inactivated (Vi) | Probably safe |
| | Live oral | Contraindicated |
| Yellow fever | Live attenuated | CD4 ≥ 500: probably safe |
| | | CD4 ≤ 200: contraindicated |

Adapted from van Gompel A *et al.*, 1997

**Preparation.** HIV-infected travellers should be advised about the possible
infectious risks and the means to prevent them. Antimicrobial prophylaxis
for travellers' diarrhoea is generally not recommended because of the
increased risk of adverse effects to medications. However, if there is a risk of
diarrhoeal illnesses, an antimicrobial agent (such as ciprofloxacin) should be
carried for empirical use. HIV-infected travellers should carry a doctor's
letter and should know where to seek medical assistance while travelling
should they need it.

**Vaccinations** that can be given to HIV-infected individuals are shown in
Table 3.4. In general, live vaccines should be avoided. A possible exception
is the measles vaccine, which is recommended for non-immune individuals;
however, the measles vaccine should be avoided in the severely
immunocompromised. In some cases, alternative inactivated vaccines are

available and should be used instead (e.g. poliomyelitis and typhoid). The safety and efficacy of yellow-fever vaccine in HIV-infected persons is uncertain; the decision to administer this vaccine must be considered on an individual basis. Inactivated vaccines should be given as they would to non-HIV-infected individuals.

CHAPTER 4

# Motion sickness and jet lag

## Motion sickness

Motion sickness is a frequently debilitating condition occasionally associated with passive transportation by sea, air and road. Characteristic symptoms and signs are nausea, vomiting, cold sweats, pallor and yawning. Given the right circumstances, virtually everyone can be affected, though it is severe in about 5% of people. The cause is incompletely understood; disturbed labyrinthine function is involved, which is probably the result of conflicting inputs to the brain from visual and labyrinthine sensors.

**Risk factors.** Women typically suffer from motion sickness more than men, and this is worse during menstruation and pregnancy. Maximum susceptibility occurs between 12 and 21 years of age, and there is also an association with migraine. Certain foods and odours, and the sound of others vomiting can accelerate the onset of symptoms.

Although changes in speed and direction can cause motion sickness, up and down movement is the most powerful inducer. Furthermore, a cycle frequency of approximately 1 per 16 seconds is the greatest stimulus, while frequencies more than one cycle per second produce little motion sickness.

**Adaptation to motion sickness.** A characteristic feature of motion sickness is the ability to habituate to the causative environmental stimuli. This adaptation is motion specific and may not necessarily transfer to different modes of transportation. For example, passengers adapted to travel on a large ship frequently get seasick when transferred to a small boat. Adaptation is lost after the stimulus has been discontinued for a few days.

**Prevention.** Several measures can be taken to help prevent or minimize motion sickness. These include:
- restricting visual activity by gazing at the horizon, minimizing fixation on close moving objects and avoiding reading; if possible, closing eyes and lying flat can be useful
- minimizing body movements

- good ventilation
- avoiding potentially noxious stimuli, large meals and alcohol
- participating in distracting activities.

While travelling by car, the best position is in the front seat, with eyes fixed on the horizon and fresh air ventilation. Motion sickness when actually driving is unusual. During air travel, the best position is between the wings. Similarly, on-board ships, a central position in a mid-deck is recommended.

Applying acupressure to the wrist with commercially available wristbands has no proven efficacy.

**Drug prophylaxis.** Many drugs have been used in an attempt to prevent motion sickness. Antihistamines and phenothiazines are the most popular (Table 4.1). Both may produce anticholinergic side-effects, particularly drowsiness, which can be problematic.

## Jet lag

Jet lag, or circadian dyschronism, occurs following rapid flight across several time zones. It is particularly common after time-zone changes of more than

TABLE 4.1

**Drugs most frequently used for motion sickness prophylaxis**

| Medication | Dose | Duration of protective effect |
|---|---|---|
| Cinnarizine and domperidone | 20 mg 15 mg | 4 hours Second dose after 4 hours |
| Cyclizine | 50 mg | > 4 hours |
| Dimenhydrinate and caffeine | 50 mg 50 mg | 4 hours |
| Ginger root | 250 mg | 4 hours Second dose after 4 hours |
| Meclozine and caffeine | 12.5 mg 10 mg | 12 hours |
| Cinnarizine | 25 mg | > 6 hours Second dose the following morning |
| Scopolamine | 0.5 mg patch | 72 hours |

From Schmid R *et al*, 1994

5 hours. Characteristic symptoms include fatigue, loss of concentration and an inability to sleep at the new night-time. Headache and gastrointestinal disturbances are also frequently experienced. Jet lag can occasionally have major consequences, particularly if the sufferer is someone who needs to perform at a high level shortly after arrival in the new time zone, such as a businessman or athlete.

Symptoms worsen as more time zones are crossed; it is also possible that they are more acute in the elderly. Eastward flights are generally associated with greater sleep disruption than westward ones. Moreover, adjustment to the new time zone tends to be slower after eastward flights – about 1 hour per day – than after westward flights (1.5 hours per day).

**Prevention** measures include those that:
- minimize the amount of jet lag experienced
- alleviate the symptoms of jet lag when they develop
- promote body clock adjustment to the new time zone.

The latter applies only to stays of longer than 3 days.

*Pre-travel countermeasures* include adding a stopover of a day or so to a journey, which results in less severe jet lag, and getting a full night's sleep for 2–3 days before departure. Avoid important activities immediately after arrival at the new time zone if possible. Watches should be set to the new time zone on departure, and eating and sleeping times adjusted accordingly.

*On arrival,* travellers should be advised to:
- try to sleep at the local time
- take naps of less than 1 hour during the adjustment time; naps are important for topping up total sleep time and improving alertness, but if longer than 1 hour (particularly if during the night of the departure time zone) can retard adjustment to the new time zone and increase the risk of sleep inertia (a transient period of depressed performance immediately after waking)
- minimize alcohol consumption
- expose themselves to sunlight or other bright light to aid adjustment.

### Treatment

*Melatonin* may have a role in both alleviating the symptoms of jet lag and promoting body-clock adjustment. Melatonin clearly relieves fatigue, and promotes sleep and alertness at the new time zone. The extent to which melatonin's effects are due to alteration of the body clock remains uncertain.

Timing of melatonin ingestion is very important, though the ideal administration times and dose are still unclear. In general, it is recommended that melatonin is taken around 20.00–22.00 h local time following arrival in a new destination for 3–4 days for both eastward and westward flights. For eastward flights, some recommend a dose at 18.00–19.00 h local time on the day of departure. Most studies of melatonin for jet lag have used doses of 5 mg, though doses of 2–3 mg have also been used.

The main side-effect is drowsiness and, consequently, activities involving driving or operating machinery should be avoided for 4–5 hours after administration. For the same reason, improper timing of administration after arrival at a new destination may adversely affect performance. Melatonin may interact with other hormones and should therefore be avoided in pregnancy and given with caution to prepubertal children.

*Other hypnotics.* Benzodiazepines may help promote sleep during the first 2–3 nights in a new time zone. However, they have not been shown to assist body-clock adjustment, and may have residual detrimental effects on alertness and psychomotor performance. In general, benzodiazepines should only be used when other measures are ineffective, and should be taken at the lowest effective dose. Drugs with shorter half-lives may have less residual effects.

CHAPTER 5
# Vaccines

Childhood vaccination programmes, recommendations for travel vaccines and availability of specific vaccine preparations vary considerably around the world. Moreover, regional disease risks change with time. Although this chapter serves as an overview of vaccines available to travellers, it is essential that local sources be consulted at the time of travel (see Appendix A). Contraindications to vaccination and risks of adverse events should also be discussed with individuals. A summary of vaccination information is provided in Table 5.1 and should be considered broadly applicable guidelines for most countries.

## Cholera

Cholera rarely affects travellers. The currently available vaccines have limited effects and short durations of action, and are not recommended for travellers. A parenteral, inactivated whole-cell vaccine is widely available, but is virtually obsolete; a more immunogenic, live attenuated, oral cholera vaccine is available in some countries, including Canada, Europe and Latin America. Further development of oral vaccines is underway to increase their efficacy in children and their duration of protection. Such vaccines would be useful for aid workers and other personnel working in communities with a high prevalence of cholera. Currently available oral vaccines are most promising in controlling cholera outbreaks, particularly in discrete communities such as refugee camps. At the time of publication, no country requires cholera vaccination as a condition of entry. However, some local authorities occasionally require documentation, and a single dose is usually sufficient to satisfy these requirements.

## Diphtheria

Diphtheria is very rare in individuals who have received both the primary immunization course and the reinforcing vaccine doses recommended in later childhood. However, recent outbreaks suggest that immunity may decline with time. Children and adults who have not been immunized should be vaccinated prior to travel, and adults immunized more than 10 years previously should be offered a booster dose. The adult diphtheria vaccine is now combined with tetanus toxoid.

### *Haemophilus influenzae* type b

The *Haemophilus influenzae* type b (Hib) vaccine should be available to all children under 5 years of age for whom travel advice is sought, and who have not already received it as part of their vaccination programme. It is not recommended routinely at other ages, but should be considered in individuals with lymphoreticular or haematopoietic malignancy, antibody dyscrasia, asplenia, bone marrow transplantation or HIV infection.

### Hepatitis A

Inactivated hepatitis A virus vaccine is recommended for travel to areas with high transmission rates (see Chapter 11). Several inactivated hepatitis A vaccines are currently available, including Havrix® (SmithKline Beecham), VAQTA® (Merck), AVAXIM® (Pasteur Merieux MSD) and Epaxal Berna® (Berna), all of which are safe and very effective. A single dose prior to travel affords protection for 6–12 months. A booster 6–12 months later extends protection for probably more than 10 years. It is recommended that the booster vaccine should be the same vaccine (i.e. produced by the same manufacturer) as the primary dose. However, preliminary data suggest that Havrix and VAQTA may be used interchangeably. A combined hepatitis A and hepatitis B vaccine, Twinrix®, and a combined hepatitis A and typhoid vaccine, Hepatyrix® (SmithKline Beecham), are also available.

### Hepatitis A immune globulin (gamma globulin)

With the availability of effective hepatitis A vaccines, immune globulin is limited largely to travellers seeking advice less than 2 weeks before departure as the active vaccine immune response takes 4 weeks. If the active vaccine is administered less than 2 weeks before departure, immune globulin can be given simultaneously to give protection until antibodies reach protective levels. This results in lower peak antibody levels than if the vaccine was given alone, but protective levels from the active vaccination last for 6 months, after which a booster can be given.

TABLE 5.1

## Vaccine information for travel

| Vaccine | Type | Route of administration | Primary series |
|---------|------|------------------------|----------------|
| Cholera<br>– parenteral<br>– live oral | Inactivated<br>Live attenuated | sc or im<br>po | Two doses 1 week or more apart<br>One dose |
| Diphtheria/<br>tetanus | Toxoid | im | Three doses at 0, 1–2<br>and 6–12 months |
| *Haemophilus influenzae* b | Protein–polysaccharide conjugate | im | Three doses at 0, 1<br>and 6 months |
| Hepatitis A<br>– Havrix® 1440<br>  EL U/ml | Inactivated | im | One dose |
| – Havrix® 720<br>  EL U/ml | Inactivated | im | Two doses at 0 and<br>30 days |
| – VAQTA® | Inactivated | im | One dose |
| – Immune<br>  globulin | Pooled<br>immunoglobulin | im | One dose |
| Hepatitis A+B<br>(Twinrix®) | Inactivated (A) +<br>recombinant protein B | im | Three doses at 0, 1<br>and 6 months |
| Hepatitis B | Recombinant hepatitis B<br>surface antigen protein | im | Three doses at 0, 1<br>and 6 months OR<br>four doses at 0, 1, 2<br>and 12 months OR 0, 7, 21<br>days and 12 months |
| Hepatitis A +<br>typhoid vaccine<br>(Hepatyrix®) | Havrix® 1440 EL U/ml<br>+ 25 µg Vi *S. typhi*<br>polysaccharide in 1 ml | im | Single dose followed by booster<br>of Hepatyrix® or hepatitis A<br>vaccine at 6–12 months |
| Influenza | Inactivated | im | One dose |
| Japanese<br>encephalitis | Inactivated | sc | Three doses at 0, 1<br>and 3–4 weeks |
| Lyme disease | Recombinant outer<br>membrane protein | im | Three doses at 0, 1<br>and 12 months |
| Measles | Live attenuated | im or sc | Single dose (booster required<br>at 12–15 months if less than<br>12 months at time of vaccination) |
| Measles/<br>mumps/rubella | Live attenuated | im or sc | Single dose, booster<br>in children |

| Booster interval | Efficacy | Lower age limit | Comments |
|---|---|---|---|
| 6 months | 50% | 6 months | Not currently recommended |
| 6 months | 80% | 2 years | Oral vaccine not recommended in pregnancy or if immunosuppressed |
| 10 years | 80–99% | 2 months | |
| None | 95% | 2 months | |
| 6–12 months (then protection for at least 10 years) | 98% | 2 years | If possible, avoid in pregnancy |
| 3 months (2 ml dose) or 5 months (5 ml dose) | | 0 | |
| As for individual components | Probably > 90% | 2 years | If possible, avoid in pregnancy |
| 3 years | 90% | – | Healthcare and aid workers, and high-risk groups |
| Further boosters as for individual components | As for components | 15 years | If possible, avoid in pregnancy |
| 1 year | 70% | 6 months | May be used in pregnancy |
| 3 years | 95% | 1 year | Not recommended in pregnancy |
| Data not available | 78% | 15 years | Not recommended in pregnancy |
| None | 90% | 6 months | Not recommended in pregnancy or if immunosuppressed |
| None | 90% | 12 months | Not recommended in pregnancy or if immunosuppressed |

TABLE 5.1 (continued)

| Vaccine | Type | Route of administration | Primary series |
|---|---|---|---|
| Meningococcal A, C, Y, W135 or A+C | Polysaccharide | sc or im | One dose |
| Meningococcal C | Protein–polysaccharide conjugate | im or sc | One dose (three doses at 1 month intervals if under 1 year) |
| Pertussis – whole cell – acellular | Whole cell Purified protein | im | Three doses in infancy |
| Pneumococcal | 23-valent polysaccharide | sc or im | Single dose |
| | 7-valent protein– polysaccharide conjugate | im or sc | Three doses in infancy; single dose at other ages |
| Poliomyelitis – oral (OPV) – inactivated (IPV) | Live attenuated Inactivated | po im or sc | Both vaccines: three doses at 0, 1–2 and 6–12 months (adults), but IPV preferred |
| Rabies | Inactivated | im or id (HDCV) | Three doses at 0, 7 and 21/28 days |
| Tetanus – see diphtheria/tetanus | | | |
| Tick-borne encephalitis | Inactivated | im | Two doses at 0 and 1 month |
| Tuberculosis (BCG) | Live attenuated | id | One dose |
| Typhoid – inactivated parenteral – capsular Vi – oral Ty21a | Inactivated Polysaccharide Live attenuated | sc im po | Two doses ≥ 4 weeks apart One dose One capsule every 2 days (four doses) |
| Varicella | Live attenuated | sc | One dose |
| Yellow fever | Live attenuated | sc | One dose |

id, intradermal; im, intramuscular; po, oral; sc, subcutaneous

| Booster interval | Efficacy | Lower age limit | Comments |
|---|---|---|---|
| None | > 70% | 2 years | |
| None | Unknown | 0 | New vaccine for endemic disease available in the UK |
| ? 10 years | 80% | 2 months | |
| 5 years | 70% | 2 years | |
| Unknown | > 90% | 0 | Now available for routine infant immunization in the USA: imminent licensure anticipated in Canada |
| 10 years | 99% | 2 months | If possible, avoid OPV in pregnancy |
| 10 years | 99% | 2 months | |
| 3 years | 99% | 0 | If possible, avoid in pregnancy |
| 1 year | Unknown | | If possible, avoid in pregnancy |
| None | ? | 0 | If possible, avoid in pregnancy |
| 3 years | 50–80% | 6 months | Oral Ty21a not recommended in pregnancy or if immunosuppressed |
| 2 years | | 2 years | |
| 5 years | | 6 years | |
| None | > 90% | 12 months | Not recommended in pregnancy or if immunosuppressed |
| 10 years | 99% | 9 months | If possible, avoid in pregnancy |

## Hepatitis B

Hepatitis B vaccine is recommended for:

- all healthcare workers
- aid workers travelling to areas of high endemicity
- individuals from high-risk groups
- individuals who plan to reside permanently in areas of high endemicity (see Chapter 11).

The vaccine comprises hepatitis B surface antigen, and about 95% of vaccine recipients seroconvert after the standard primary three-dose series. An accelerated schedule for travellers with less than 6 months before the date of travel, the time needed for the standard series, has received approval from the Food and Drink Administration (FDA) in the USA. This consists of three doses given at 0, 1 and 2 months, with a booster dose at 12 months.

## Influenza

Several recent outbreaks of influenza amongst travellers have highlighted the importance of offering this vaccine to high-risk individuals (see Chapter 11). A single-dose vaccine is administered each year.

## Japanese encephalitis

Japanese encephalitis vaccine is recommended for travellers staying more than 1 month in endemic areas or for shorter periods in very high-risk areas (see Chapter 7). Primary immunization consists of three doses given at 0, 1 and 3–4 weeks. For continuing exposure, a booster dose should be given after 3 years. Constitutional symptoms occur in approximately 20% of vaccine recipients and severe allergic reactions in 0.6%. A promising Chinese live attenuated virus vaccine is highly efficacious after two doses, but further safety data are required.

## Lyme disease

Travellers to highly endemic areas who plan to hike, camp or work in forested areas or meadows are at greatest risk (see Chapter 10). A new recombinant lipoprotein vaccine that consists of a surface protein (OspA) of the causative organism *Borrelia burgdorferi* has recently become available in North America. After three doses at 0, 1 and 12 months, efficacy in North

America is 78%; efficacy elsewhere is unclear. Constitutional symptoms occur in 1% of recipients. Safety and immunogenicity data for children are awaited.

## Measles, mumps and rubella

The measles, mumps and rubella (MMR) vaccine is available to children in many countries as part of the primary immunization strategy. Most adults who grew up prior to vaccine introduction have naturally acquired immunity. Adult immunity varies from country to country, as the measles vaccine was introduced at different times around the world; there is a group of adults that neither received the vaccine nor had the infection during childhood.

Measles vaccine is recommended for non-immune individuals travelling to endemic areas. A single dose should be offered to unvaccinated adults and children, and to adults who received only one dose of MMR in childhood. MMR or measles vaccine can immunize against measles even if the recipient is already immune to rubella and mumps. Infants over 6 months of age, but who are too young to have received their first dose of MMR vaccine (< 12 months), should receive measles vaccine before travelling to an endemic area. They will need a booster dose at 12–15 months.

## Meningococcal disease

Travellers to areas where epidemic meningococcal disease (see Chapter 11) is prevalent should be advised to receive a single dose of meningococcal vaccine containing A, C, Y and W135 polysaccharide or A+C if the tetravalent vaccine is unavailable. There is currently no vaccine against serogroup B. This vaccine induces protective antibody against the serogroups in the vaccine, but immunological evidence of protection is relatively short-lived (3 years). Responses are reduced in early childhood and decline more rapidly. Primary immunization consists of a single dose that affords immunity for 3–4 years.

A new highly effective vaccine against serogroup C meningococcal disease became available in the UK in October 1999. It consists of a protein C–polysaccharide conjugate, which greatly enhances the immunogenicity of the vaccine and produces high levels of persisting antibody even in infants, and is currently being used for routine immunization of children in the UK.

Serogroup C meningococcal disease has not been a problem among travellers, and this vaccine is not generally administered. However, it is advisable in individuals at risk of meningococcal disease, such as those with complement deficiency or hyposplenism. Data are available for a serogroup A meningococcal protein–polysaccharide vaccine that would be valuable for those working in endemic areas who require long-term protection. This vaccine is not yet widely available. Early trials of a serogroup Y protein–polysaccharide conjugate vaccine are also in progress.

Most cases of meningococcal disease in industrialized nations are caused by serogroup B meningococci, for which no vaccine is currently available, though clinical trials are ongoing. Although hyperendemic disease caused by both B and C strains is reported around the world, the incidence in most areas remains so low that routine vaccination could not be recommended, except in exceptional circumstances.

### Pertussis

The aim of pertussis vaccination is to prevent severe infection in infants. Acellular pertussis vaccine is more immunogenic and less reactogenic than the whole cell vaccine and is used as standard in many countries. An accelerated schedule can be given to non-immune infants who are due to travel (three doses, 1 month apart as used in the UK accelerated schedule), starting at 2 months of age. For non-immune older children and adults, the benefits of vaccination are less clear as the condition is usually mild. However, vaccinating non-immune parents and siblings may prevent transmission from them to non-immune young infants. Outbreaks of pertussis have recently been reported among adults in England, Canada, The Netherlands and the USA, and have resulted in disease in susceptible infant contacts.

### Pneumococcal

The 23-valent pneumococcal polysaccharide vaccine is not routinely recommended for travel, but a single dose should be considered routine in high-risk groups such as those with hyposplenism, chronic heart, lung or liver disease, diabetes mellitus, sickle cell disease, coeliac disease, HIV infection and other immunosuppression. The vaccine may be offered to adults over 65 years of age because of the increased incidence of infection in this group. A single dose confers protection for about 5 years. A new 7-valent conjugate vaccine that could eventually replace the currently available vaccine was licensed in the USA in 2000 and appears highly effective in infants for protection against invasive pneumococcal disease caused by vaccine serotypes.

## Poliomyelitis

Routine vaccination against polio exists worldwide, and eradication of polio is anticipated in the near future (see Chapter 8). Any unimmunized adult or child should be offered vaccination with three doses of either inactivated poliomyelitis vaccine (IPV) or oral poliomyelitis vaccine (OPV). IPV should be used for the immunosuppressed. An additional dose can be offered to individuals, typically healthcare and aid workers in Asia and Africa, travelling to discrete endemic areas.

## Rabies

Rabies is universally fatal, and safe vaccine and immunoglobulin for post-exposure prophylaxis cannot be guaranteed in all countries. Furthermore, vaccines in many non-industrialized countries are prepared directly from neural tissue rather than cell culture and have a higher incidence of adverse effects. Pre-exposure rabies vaccination is therefore recommended for travellers to endemic areas who are at high risk of exposure to a rabid animal. Rabies vaccination is also recommended for laboratory workers handling the virus, veterinarians, animal control and wildlife workers, healthcare workers, cave explorers (risk of exposure to bats) and backpackers travelling to areas where medical care is limited.

Several types of inactivated rabies vaccine are available for both pre-exposure immunization and post-exposure prophylaxis, including:

- human diploid cell vaccine (HDCV)
- rabies vaccine adsorbed (RVA)
- purified chick embryo cell vaccine (PCEC).

All are given intramuscularly (1 ml dose). HDCV can also be given intradermally (0.1 ml dose), though this is less efficacious with concurrent administration of chloroquine. Pre-exposure prophylaxis consists of three doses given on days 0, 7 and 21 (or day 28). Post-exposure prophylaxis is considered in Chapter 11.

## Tetanus

*Clostridium tetani* is found worldwide. All unimmunized travellers should be advised to receive three doses of tetanus toxoid. Previously immunized travellers should be advised to receive a reinforcing dose of vaccine if 10 years have elapsed since either their primary course or last booster dose (5 years is recommended in some countries). Some authorities do not recommend further booster doses when five doses of vaccine have been administered unless there has been a tetanus-prone injury.

## Tick-borne encephalitis

An inactivated whole-cell vaccine is available for travellers at risk for tick-borne encephalitis (see Chapter 10). Two doses of vaccine are offered 1–3 months apart to confer 12 months' protection. A third dose is recommended after 9–12 months for those with continuing exposure. Following three doses, the protection rate is more than 98% and lasts for 3–5 years. Several more rapid vaccination schedules have shown similar efficacy. Side-effects are infrequent, and are most commonly reactions at the injection site. Egg allergy is a relative contraindication to administration.

## Tuberculosis

Recommendations for primary immunization of children with bacillus Calmette-Guérin (BCG) vaccine vary around the world. The vaccine is used routinely for childhood vaccination in the UK, but not in North America. Efficacy studies have not clearly demonstrated that the vaccine provides useful protection, though it probably affords reasonable protection against miliary tuberculosis and tuberculous meningitis in infants and children. BCG vaccine may be considered for travellers who plan to spend more than 1 month in endemic areas, and for those who expect to have close contact with people with tuberculosis (see Chapter 11).

## Typhoid

Typhoid is endemic in Africa, Asia, Central and South America, Haiti and Iran (see Chapter 8). Avoiding contaminated water and food is the most important way of preventing typhoid. Vaccination is recommended for travellers to high-risk areas where sanitation and hygiene are likely to be poor, and who will have prolonged exposure to potentially contaminated food and water.

Three types of typhoid vaccine are available (Table 5.1):

* heat phenol-inactivated whole-cell parenteral vaccine, which has been the mainstay for many years, but has been superseded by newer preparations
* capsular Vi polysaccharide vaccine, which is administered parenterally
* oral live attenuated vaccine, which is manufactured from the Ty21a strain of *Salmonella typhi*.

Side-effects are particularly common with the inactivated parenteral vaccine, with 7–24% of recipients experiencing fever, 1.5–3.0% headache, and 3–35% pain and swelling at the injection site. Consequently, unless contraindicated, the oral Ty21a or parenteral Vi vaccine is preferred, though the Vi vaccine is poorly immunogenic in early childhood. New protein–polysaccharide conjugate vaccines are currently being evaluated in this age group.

Oral Ty21a vaccine capsules need to be kept refrigerated and should not be administered simultaneously with antibacterial agents or mefloquine. Simultaneous administration of chloroquine or immune globulin does not seem to be a problem, and immunogenicity does not appear to be affected by concurrent administration of live viral vaccines.

## Varicella

A live virus vaccine against chickenpox is available in many countries and has recently been introduced into the primary immunization strategy in the USA. Some authorities have recommended it for travellers with no history of infection or vaccination.

## Yellow fever

Yellow-fever vaccine (see Chapter 7 and Appendix A) is recommended for people who.

* travel or live in infected areas or rural areas within endemic zones
* travel to countries that require a yellow fever vaccination certificate
* visit yellow fever-infected countries and then travel to countries with a vaccination requirement.

Several countries, such as India, Singapore and Malaysia, do not have yellow fever but have potential vectors for the virus. Consequently, vaccination is a requirement in travellers arriving from endemic areas. Up-to-date information can be obtained from the WHO (www.who.int/ith/english/country.htm) or the Centers for Disease Control and Prevention (www.cdc.gov/travel/yelfever.htm).

Yellow-fever vaccine is extremely safe and effective. A single subcutaneous 0.5 ml dose produces seroconversion rates of more than 95% and immunity for at least 10 years (possibly lifelong). A booster dose is recommended every 10 years for those returning to or staying in endemic areas. Reactions to the vaccine are uncommon and typically mild; 2–5% report minor symptoms, including myalgia, low-grade fever or headache. Encephalitis as a complication of vaccination is rare and occurs exclusively in young children (particularly those under 3 months of age). Hypersensitivity reactions are also uncommon. As the vaccine contains egg protein, a history of egg allergy is usually regarded as a contraindication for vaccination. In reality, those with a history of anaphylactic reactions to eggs are at greatest risk, with most others usually tolerating the vaccine. A skin test can help determine whether or not the patient will tolerate the vaccine. Infants under 4 months should not receive the vaccine because of the increased risk of side-effects. Vaccination between 4 and 9 months should be given if travel to an endemic area is unavoidable. Infants over 9 months should be vaccinated if they are travelling to endemic areas. Yellow-fever vaccine should be avoided during pregnancy unless travel to a high-risk area is unavoidable.

*Timing.* Because of possible interactions, yellow-fever vaccine should ideally be administered at least 4 weeks apart from other live vaccines. If time does not permit this spacing, the vaccines can be given within this time period.

*Administration* is by certified centres only. For official purposes, the vaccine is valid 10 days after administration, and appropriate documentation should be completed on an *International Certificate of Vaccination Against Yellow Fever* at the time of vaccination. If administration of the yellow-fever vaccine is contraindicated, the traveller should carry a physician's letter (on letterhead stationery) stating that the vaccine is contraindicated for medical reasons.

CHAPTER 6
# Malaria

Malaria is caused by four protozoan species: *Plasmodium falciparum*, *Plasmodium vivax*, *Plasmodium ovale* and *Plasmodium malariae*. Transmission occurs via the bite of *Anopheles* mosquitoes and by blood transfusion. Each year, more than 200 million new cases of malaria occur in nearly 100 countries, mainly in children, and up to 3 million die. The risk to travellers varies considerably from region to region because of differences in transmission intensity, itineraries and type of travel. For example, travellers to Africa often spend considerable time (including evenings and night-time) in rural areas where the risk of malaria is high. In contrast, many travellers to Asia spend much of their time in low-risk urban areas and resorts.

## Epidemiology

Malaria is prevalent throughout the tropics and sub-tropics (Figure 6.1; see Appendix B). Country-specific information about malaria risk can be obtained from www.cdc.gov/ncidod/publications/brochures/malaria.htm, www.cdc.gov/travel/index.htm and www.who.int/ctd/html/malaria.html.

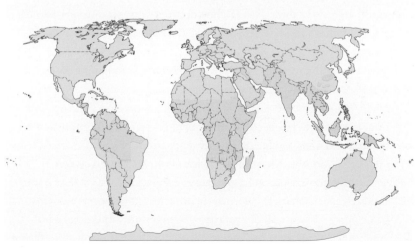

**Figure 6.1** Malaria-affected areas. Adapted from Centers for Disease Control and Prevention, 1997.

Malaria transmission varies greatly between and within countries. Some destinations within malarious countries will be malaria-free. Malaria is rarely transmitted above 1500 m altitude and is unusual in the large cities of South America and South-East Asia. However, transmission persists in urban areas of India, Pakistan, Bangladesh and parts of Africa. Local advice and region-specific advice within countries should be sought before travel and is beyond the scope of this book.

Chloroquine-resistant *P. falciparum* malaria occurs in the majority of these areas, the greatest risk being in Africa, South-East Asia and Oceania. Mefloquine-resistant malaria occurs primarily in Cambodia, Thailand and Myanmar, but has also been seen in west Africa. Resistance to sulfadoxine–pyrimethamine (Fansidar®) is common in South-East Asia and South America, and is increasing in Africa. Chloroquine-resistant *P. vivax* has been reported in Papua New Guinea, Irian Jaya, Sumatra, Myanmar, Vanuatu and India. Clinically significant resistance to *P. ovale* and *P. malariae* has not been described.

## Life cycle

Following an anopheline mosquito bite, malarial sporozoites are released into the blood, from which they preferentially invade hepatocytes (Figure 6.2). Following a period of division, merozoites are released into the circulation after 7–21 days. *P. vivax* however may not produce merozoites for up to 2 months, and both *P. vivax* and *P. ovale* can persist within hepatocytes for years.

*P. malariae* probably does not have a persistent liver phase, but disease recrudescence may occur many years later, possibly a result of persistent low-grade parasitaemia. *P. falciparum* does not produce a persistent liver infection, but malaria has been observed in children up to 12 months after a visit to a malaria area. Parasitaemia with *P. ovale* and *P. vivax* can last from a few days to 3 months. Merozoites invade erythrocytes and undergo nuclear division to produce more merozoites, which are then released into the blood to repeat the cycle. Merozoites are released from erythrocytes every 48 hours (72 hours for *P. malariae*). Sexual forms of the parasite develop during one of these cycles and are transmitted to a mosquito during a female anopheline blood meal.

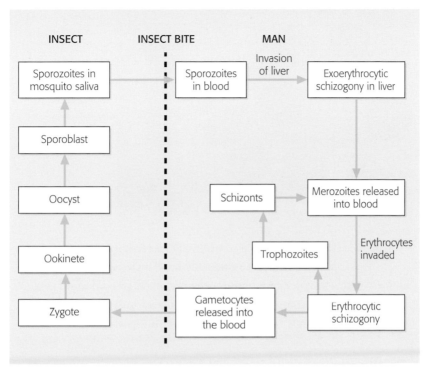

**Figure 6.2** Life cycle of a malaria parasite.

## Clinical features

The symptoms of malaria occur as merozoites are released from erythrocytes, and include fever, nausea and vomiting, and headache. Travellers should be informed about the significance of these non-specific symptoms during and after a visit to an endemic area, even when compliant with antimalarials.

Up to 2% of erythrocytes may become infected in *P. vivax* and *P. ovale*, but up to 60% may be infected in falciparum malaria (Figure 6.3). Anaemia, jaundice, hepatosplenomegaly, hypoglycaemia and delirium are also common. Relapses may occur for up to 3 months as a result of persistent parasitaemia, and have been described for up to 12 months. Longer-term relapses with *P. vivax* or *P. ovale* are usually due to release of liver-stage parasites from 3 months up to years after the initial infection. There is no liver stage for *P. falciparum*, and recrudescence usually occurs within 3 months, but has occasionally been described 12 months after infection.

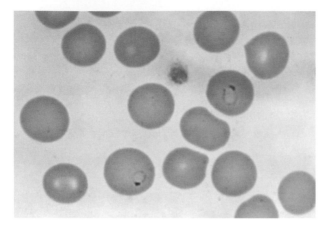

**Figure 6.3**
*Plasmodium falciparum* trophozoites in a peripheral blood smear.

Unlike the self-limited, relatively benign parasitaemia of *P. vivax* and *P. ovale*, *P. falciparum* malaria is potentially fatal in the non-immune. In addition to the non-specific symptoms, cerebral malaria (confusion, coma, high fever and convulsions), blackwater fever (haemoglobinuria and acute renal failure) and hepatic failure may occur with falciparum malaria.

## Diagnosis

Examination of a blood film by an experienced observer confirms the diagnosis. In remote areas where laboratory diagnosis is impossible, a presumptive diagnosis may be made based on the onset of unexplained fever (though this is often inaccurate). Rapid testing kits, which have performed well in the laboratory are now available for detection of the malaria antigen in blood using a 'dipstick' method. However, travellers using such kits under field conditions have failed to self-diagnose falciparum malaria. Self-testing can therefore not be recommended without careful training of the traveller.

## Prevention

At-risk travellers should be advised to take appropriate chemoprophylaxis and about personal preventative measures. They should be aware that malaria can still occur even when the best preventative measures are adhered to. Travellers should be informed that malaria can develop as soon as 6 days after initial exposure and as late as several months after leaving malarious areas. Malaria must be considered for any febrile illness that develops during or for several months after travel; medical attention should be sought promptly as a delay in diagnosis can have serious consequences.

**Personal protection** measures are at least as important as chemoprophylaxis against malaria. Measures to prevent bites include:
- avoiding exposure from dawn to dusk when anopheline mosquitoes feed
- wearing dark-coloured clothing that covers most of the body
- use of topical insect repellents on skin and clothing.

Repellents containing N,N-diethyl-meta-toluamide (DEET) are the most effective; a concentration of 30–35% is effective and gives 3–4 hours' protection. DEET has rarely been associated with neurotoxicity, and occurrences have usually been in children. Permethrin-impregnated bed nets provide additional benefit, and clothing can be sprayed with permethrin.

**Chemoprophylaxis** aims to prevent death and severe disease, but cannot prevent malarial infection. As falciparum malaria is the most severe (causing virtually all deaths due to malaria) and resistant disease, the choice of chemoprophylactic regimen is focused on the risk of malaria due to *P. falciparum*. In general, chemoprophylaxis should begin 1 week before entering a malarious area and continued for 4 weeks after leaving it. Compliance cannot be overemphasized. Non-compliance is particularly common among young adults spending more than 1 month in malarious areas.

Several drugs are currently available for antimalarial chemoprophylaxis, though some may not be available universally. The choice of regimen depends on local knowledge of malaria epidemiology and patterns of resistance (Table 6.1). The variations in national guidelines illustrate the uncertainties about risks and benefits. Some of the most widely used guidelines are those developed by the WHO and CDC. Table 6.2 incorporates features of both guidelines; variations may be required, depending on individual circumstances.

Although the combination of chloroquine and proguanil is not as effective against *P. falciparum* as either mefloquine or doxycycline, it may be used in special circumstances. This combination is still moderately effective in parts of Africa, but not in South-East Asia and Oceania. It may also be

TABLE 6.1

**Malarial risk areas***

| Risk areas | Regions | Recommended prophylactic regimen |
|---|---|---|
| Low risk of chloroquine resistance | Middle East, Central America, Mexico, Haiti, Turkey, Egypt, Mauritius | Chloroquine |
| Areas where *P. falciparum* is known to be chloroquine sensitive or mildly resistant | West Asia, Mauritius, Africa, China, Mexico, Central America, and parts of Haiti, Dominican Republic, Turkey, Egypt | Chloroquine and proguanil or mefloquine |
| Areas where *P. falciparum* is known to be chloroquine resistant | South-East Asia, Indian subcontinent, parts of tropical South America, parts of Africa, Pacific Islands and New Guinea, India, Panama | Mefloquine or doxycycline (or primaquine) |
| Mefloquine-resistant area | Thai–Cambodian border, Thai–Myanmar border | Doxycycline |

*Risk varies greatly within countries and between seasons, and local advice should be sought

the chemoprophylactic regimen of choice for those allergic to or intolerant of mefloquine and doxycycline.

**Chloroquine** alone is an acceptable antimalarial agent in areas without chloroquine resistance, namely Central America, the Caribbean and the Middle East. Chloroquine is generally well tolerated and is safe during pregnancy. Side-effects are typically minor and include gastrointestinal disturbance, headache and dizziness. Psychosis is rare. Retinal changes occur rarely, if at all, at the doses used for malaria chemoprophylaxis. Chloroquine is suitable for long-term prophylaxis.

**Mefloquine** is the most effective antimalarial chemoprophylactic at the time of press. It is highly effective against all malarial species, though resistance is emerging. Mefloquine-resistant falciparum malaria occurs around the Thai–Cambodian and Thai–Myanmar borders.

TABLE 6.2

**Chemoprophylactic doses with various agents**

| Drug | Adult dose | Paediatric dose | Duration of dosing before/after exposure |
| --- | --- | --- | --- |
| Chloroquine | 300 mg base orally weekly | 5 mg/kg orally of base weekly (max 300 mg) | 1–2/4 weeks |
| Doxycycline | 100 mg orally daily | 2 mg/kg orally daily (> 8 years only; max 100 mg) | 1 day/4 weeks |
| Mefloquine | 250 mg orally weekly (228 mg base) | < 15 kg; 5 mg/kg/week orally<br>15–19 kg; 62.5 mg (1/4 tablet)<br>20–30 kg; 125 mg (1/2 tablet)<br>31–45 kg; 187.5 mg (3/4 tablet)<br>> 45 kg; 250 mg (1 tablet) | 1–2/4 weeks |
| Proguanil | 200 mg/day orally | < 2 years; 50 mg/day<br>2–6 years; 100 mg/day<br>7–10 years; 150 mg/day<br>> 10 years; 200 mg/day | 1–2/4 weeks |
| Primaquine (not yet available for prophylaxis) | 30 mg/day base | < 2 years; 3.75 mg/day<br>2–5 years; 7.5 mg<br>6–12 years; 15 mg<br>> 12 years; 30 mg | 0/2 days |
| Malarone | 250 mg atovaquone + 100 mg proguanil daily | 11–20 kg; 62.5 mg/25 mg<br>21–30 kg; 125 mg/50 mg<br>31–40 kg; 187.5 mg/75 mg<br>> 40 kg; 250 mg/100 mg | 2/7 days |

Mefloquine is generally well tolerated, though approximately 20% of users experience minor side-effects, such as headache, nausea and vomiting, vivid dreams and dizziness. These symptoms tend to be transient and self-limiting. Of more serious concern, and the subject of considerable media attention, are the potential neuropsychiatric side-effects of mefloquine (including psychosis and convulsions). A study of European travellers revealed mefloquine and chloroquine had similar rates of serious neuropsychiatric complications, and that these rates were similar to those in the general population. Other researchers have disagreed. However, it appears that the frequency of serious side-effects has been overstated, but it is important to warn travellers that they may occur. People with a history of seizures or psychiatric disorders (particularly depression) should avoid taking mefloquine.

Mefloquine has been associated with a prolonged QT interval and asymptomatic sinus bradycardia. For this reason, mefloquine should be avoided in travellers with cardiac conduction abnormalities.

Given the long half-life of mefloquine, a loading-dose regimen (e.g. 250 mg daily for 3 days for adults) will allow a therapeutic level to be reached in about 4 days.

**Doxycycline** is as effective as mefloquine in most malarious areas, and is the preferred chemoprophylactic agent for travellers to mefloquine-resistant areas. Side-effects include nausea (particularly when taken on an empty stomach), thrush and photosensitivity reactions. It is important to warn travellers about the latter, which can be minimized by taking the drug in the evening and using sunscreens liberally. The safety of long-term use of doxycycline for malaria chemoprophylaxis is not established, though prolonged use for the treatment of acne has caused few serious problems.

**Proguanil** is usually taken in combination with chloroquine. This combination is not as effective as either mefloquine or doxycycline, but is still useful in some areas and for those who are intolerant to other agents. Proguanil is the safest antimalarial.

### Future chemoprophylactics

*Primaquine* is likely to become a major malarial chemoprophylactic in the future. Although it commonly causes gastrointestinal side-effects, these are virtually eliminated by taking the drug with food. Haemolysis occurs in patients with glucose-6-phosphate dehydrogenase deficiency (G6PD) taking primaquine. G6PD affects 10% of Africans, and is not uncommon in those originating from the Mediterranean and Asia. The haemolysis may be fatal and is more severe in non-Africans with G6PD. Before using primaquine, G6PD should be excluded.

*Atovaquone/proguanil (Malarone™).* Fixed-dose combination tablets of atovaquone and proguanil have recently become available in some countries. The preparation is available as both 250 mg atovaquone/100 mg proguanil hydrochloride (adult dose) and 62.5 mg atovaquone/25 mg proguanil hydrochloride (paediatric dose) tablets. Although experience with this drug for chemoprophylaxis in non-immune travellers is limited, trials have found it to be effective and well tolerated.

*Azithromycin* is also a potential prophylactic, but it has only limited efficacy against *P. falciparum*. Further data are required before azithromycin can be recommended.

**Vaccines.** There are currently no vaccines for malaria, though efforts to develop them are intense. Recent initiatives to examine vaccine candidates and the availability of the *Plasmodium* genome are likely to accelerate progress in the next few years. A number of approaches are under evaluation, since the disappointing trials of Patarroyo's SPf66 synthetic peptide vaccine. Progress is hampered by the complex nature of the organism, limited knowledge about important immune mechanisms and targets for immunity, antigenic variation and diversity, and absence of good *in vitro* correlates of immunity. Current research is examining multi-stage, multi-antigen vaccines to target antigens expressed during multiple stages of the parasite's life cycle. Liver- and blood stage DNA vaccines are also undergoing investigation and may be combined in a DNA/recombinant protein vaccine in the future. Although the aim of vaccine development is to prevent infection with malaria parasites, a reasonable goal for those living in malaria endemic regions is a reduction in disease severity and prevention of life-threatening cerebral malaria or anaemia.

**Emergency self-treatment (EST)**, or emergency standby treatment, refers to the self-administration of antimalarials in situations in which malaria is suspected and medical assistance is unavailable. EST should be followed by medical consultation as soon as possible.

Although unnecessary for most travellers, EST may be indicated for certain individuals. These individuals include:

- long-term travellers or residents in malarious areas who either cannot or do not want to take long-term chemoprophylaxis
- travellers whose exposure to malarious areas is brief, including aircrew, business people and others who make frequent short-term trips to areas with a low risk of malaria
- travellers at high risk for falciparum malaria who are taking sub-optimal or no chemoprophylaxis.

Whenever EST is contemplated, it is essential that sufficient time is spent with the traveller explaining the pros and cons of EST and giving instructions about when and how to administer it. Rapid immunochromatographic tests for the diagnosis of malaria that utilize finger-prick blood samples are available and may assist self-diagnosis. As yet, they have not been adequately studied in travellers.

*Chloroquine* is appropriate only for areas with chloroquine-sensitive malaria (Table 6.3).

TABLE 6.3

**Doses for chloroquine emergency self-treatment**

| Weight (kg) | Age (years) | Number of tablets 100 mg base | | | 150 mg base | | |
| | | Day 1 | Day 2 | Day 3 | Day 1 | Day 2 | Day 3 |
|---|---|---|---|---|---|---|---|
| 5–6 | < 4 months | 0.5 | 0.5 | 0.5 | 0.5 | 0.25 | 0.25 |
| 7–10 | 4–11 months | 1 | 1 | 0.5 | 0.5 | 0.5 | 0.5 |
| 11–14 | 1–2 | 1.5 | 1.5 | 0.5 | 1 | 1 | 0.5 |
| 15–18 | 3–4 | 2 | 2 | 0.5 | 1 | 1 | 1 |
| 19–24 | 5–7 | 2.5 | 2.5 | 1 | 1.5 | 1.5 | 1 |
| 25–35 | 8–10 | 3.5 | 3.5 | 2 | 2.5 | 2.5 | 1 |
| 36–50 | 11–13 | 5 | 5 | 2.5 | 3 | 3 | 2 |
| 50+ | 14+ | 6 | 6 | 3 | 4 | 4 | 2 |

*Sulfadoxine–pyrimethamine (Fansidar®)* is the EST recommended by the CDC. It is well-tolerated and effective in east Africa, the Indian subcontinent and parts of Indonesia (Table 6.4).

TABLE 6.4

**Doses for sulfadoxine–pyrimethamine emergency self-treatment**

| Weight (kg) | Number of tablets (each containing 500 mg sulfadoxine and 25 mg pyrimethamine) |
|---|---|
| 5–10 | 0.5 |
| 11–20 | 1.0 |
| 21–30 | 1.5 |
| 31–45 | 2.0 |
| > 45 | 3.0 |

*Mefloquine* is not recommended by some authorities because of the high risk of adverse reactions with treatment doses. Neurological side-effects (including dizziness, lightheadedness and poor concentration) are about 60 times more likely to occur after treatment than with prophylaxis. Mefloquine EST can be given as a single dose in areas without significant mefloquine resistance or in split doses in areas with mefloquine resistance (Table 6.5).

TABLE 6.5

**Doses for mefloquine emergency self-treatment**

| Weight (kg) | Age (years) | Single dose (number of 250 mg tablets) | Split dose (number of 250 mg tablets) | |
|---|---|---|---|---|
| | | | Dose 1 | Dose 2 |
| 5–6 | 3 months | 0.25 | 0.25 | 0.25 |
| 7–8 | 4–7 months | 0.5 | 0.5 | 0.25 |
| 9–12 | 8–23 months | 0.75 | 0.75 | 0.5 |
| 13–16 | 2–3 | 1 | 1 | 0.5 |
| 17–24 | 4–7 | 1.5 | 1.5 | 1 |
| 25–35 | 8–10 | 2 | 2 | 1.5 |
| 36–50 | 11–13 | 3 | 3 | 2 |
| 51–59 | 14–15 | 3.5 | 3.5 | 2 |
| 60+ | 15+ | 4 | 4 | 2 |

*Quinine* is rarely given for EST because of the risk of adverse effects and reduced efficacy in some parts of the world. In areas where malarial parasites are susceptible to quinine, the EST dose is quinine 8 mg base/kg orally three times daily for 7 days.

*Atovaquone–proguanil (Malarone®)* is not widely available, but has shown promising results for the treatment of falciparum malaria. Atovaquone–proguanil is well-tolerated and may become a preferred EST in areas of chloroquine resistance (Table 6.6).

TABLE 6.6

**Doses for atovaquone–proguanil emergency self-treatment**

| Weight (kg) | Daily dose for 3 consecutive days* |
|---|---|
| 11–20 | 1 |
| 21–30 | 2 |
| 31–40 | 3 |
| > 40 | 4 |

*Each tablet contains 250 mg atovaquone and 100 mg proguanil

### Treatment

*Falciparum malaria* is a life-threatening illness. Travellers should be advised about the non-specific features of early malaria, to think of malaria when they are unwell and to seek help promptly. Treatment recommendations are outlined in Figure 6.4, but specialist advice should be sought. Table 6.1 outlines the areas where chloroquine resistance is common. In fact, most regions of the world have some chloroquine-resistant parasites, and local knowledge is important in guiding initial therapy in complicated malaria. In complicated falciparum malaria, resistance should be assumed when commencing empirical therapy if detailed local information is unavailable.

*Non-falciparum malaria* can usually be treated with chloroquine, followed by primaquine to kill the hypnozoites in the liver (vivax and ovale; see Figure 6.5). In some regions (Papua New Guinea, Irian Jaya, Sumatra, Myanmar, Vanuatu and India), chloroquine-resistant *P. vivax* occurs and here mefloquine or quinine plus primaquine are recommended. Primaquine

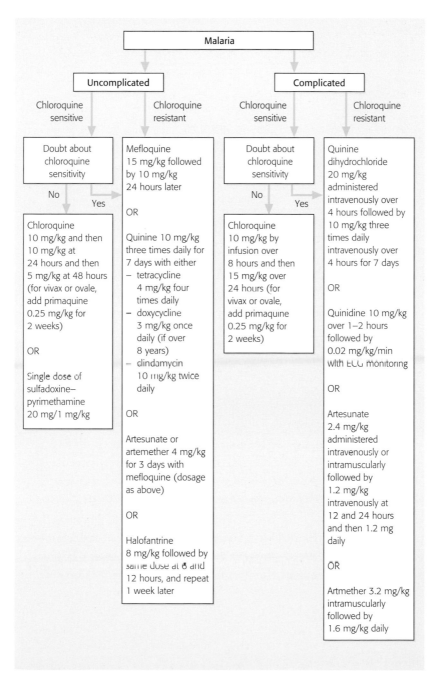

**Figure 6.4** Treatment regimens for falciparum malaria.

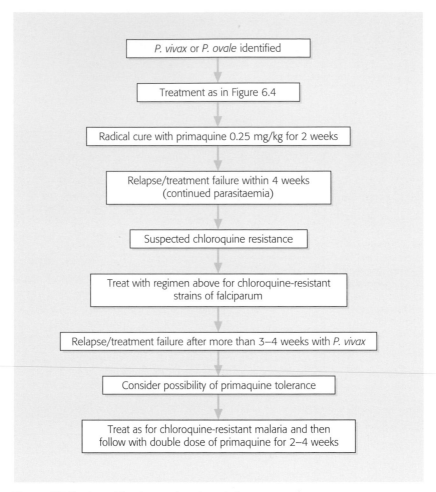

**Figure 6.5** Treatment for vivax and ovale malaria.

tolerance has been reported for *P. vivax* and should be suspected when vivax malaria recrudesces after 3–4 weeks despite adequate treatment. Higher doses and longer durations of primaquine therapy have been successful.

CHAPTER 7
# Other mosquito-transmitted diseases

There are over 3000 species of mosquito worldwide; only Antarctica and extreme altitudes (> 5500 m) are mosquito-free. In addition to being a biting nuisance, many species transmit infections to humans. Indeed, the distribution of these infections is largely determined by the presence of suitable mosquito vectors. Apart from malaria, the mosquito-transmitted infections most relevant to travellers are yellow fever, dengue and Japanese encephalitis. Mosquitoes are also vectors of many other arboviral infections and filariasis.

## Yellow fever

Yellow fever is an acute viral infection of varying severity. Although frequently asymptomatic, typical illness is characterized by the sudden onset of fever, chills, headache, nausea, vomiting and musculoskeletal pain. The incubation period is 3–6 days. Many cases then progress to a haemorrhagic phase with gastrointestinal bleeding, epistaxis, jaundice, hepatic and renal failure. Of those with jaundice, the case-fatality rate is approximately 50%. There is no effective specific therapy, and management is supportive. Recovery from yellow fever is followed by lasting immunity, and second attacks are unknown.

**Epidemiology.** Yellow-fever virus is endemic in two geographical areas, central Africa and northern South America (Figure 7.1). The virus is not present elsewhere, though mosquitoes capable of transmitting yellow fever exist outside endemic areas, in countries such as India, Singapore and Malaysia. Consequently, many countries require yellow-fever vaccination certificates for travellers arriving from yellow-fever areas. The number of cases has increased dramatically over the past two decades. However, documented yellow fever in travellers is still relatively uncommon, which may relate in part to the widespread use of yellow-fever vaccination. In 1996, at least two travellers (both unvaccinated) died of yellow fever acquired in the Brazilian Amazon.

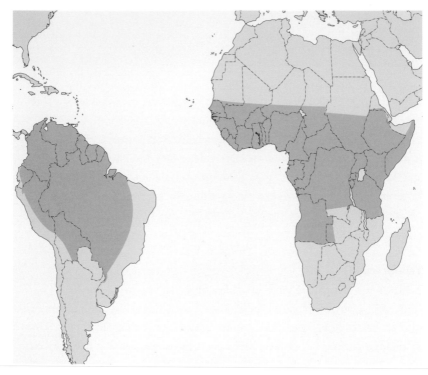

**Figure 7.1** Global distribution of yellow fever, 1996.

Several species of mosquito transmit infection to monkeys as well as humans. In Africa, the main vectors are *Aedes aegypti* and *Aedes simpsoni*, while in South America they are *Aedes aegypti* and *Haemagogus* spp. There are three possible transmission cycles for yellow fever:

- sylvatic (or jungle) yellow fever, which exists among monkeys in tropical rainforests; sporadic cases occur in humans who enter the forest
- intermediate yellow fever is found in semi-humid savannahs; semi-domestic mosquitoes infect both humans and monkeys, causing small-scale epidemics
- urban yellow fever occurs when migrants introduce the virus into densely populated areas, resulting in large epidemics.

**Prevention** is by vaccination (see Chapter 5 and Appendix A). Yellow-fever vaccine is an extremely safe and effective live attenuated vaccine. A single subcutaneous 0.5 ml dose produces seroconversion rates of more than 95%

and immunity for at least 10 years, and possibly even lifelong. A booster dose is recommended every 10 years for those returning to or staying in endemic areas.

**Recommendations.** Yellow-fever vaccination is recommended for people who:
- travel or live in infected or rural areas within yellow-fever endemic zones
- travel to countries that require a yellow-fever vaccination certificate
- visit yellow fever-infected countries and then travel to countries with a vaccination requirement.

Up-to-date information on yellow-fever vaccination requirements for individual countries is available from the WHO publication *International Travel and Health* (www.who.int/ith/english/country.htm) or the CDC's publication *Health Information for International Travel* (www.cdc.gov/travel/yelfever.htm).

## Dengue

Dengue fever is an acute febrile viral infection characterized by headache, arthralgia, myalgia and maculopapular rash, with an incubation period of 3–14 days. Although infection is typically mild and self-limiting, it may be associated with serious haemorrhagic complications and shock. Dengue haemorrhagic fever and dengue shock syndrome occur more commonly in children and in those who have previously had dengue fever. Although dengue fever is seen relatively frequently in travellers in or returning from endemic areas, severe complications are rare. Recovery from infection with one serotype provides lifelong immunity, but does not protect against the other three serotypes. Diagnosis of dengue is by serology, and treatment is supportive only.

**Epidemiology.** Dengue fever is transmitted by mosquitoes of the genus *Aedes*, particularly *A. aegypti* and *A. albopictus*. These vectors live in and around human habitation, breeding in standing water left by humans, and are most active during the day. They are present in most tropical and many sub-tropical countries (Figure 7.2). Transmission occurs in epidemics, usually during the rainy seasons.

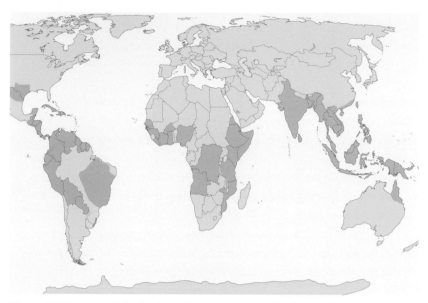

**Figure 7.2** The general distribution of dengue fever and/or dengue haemorrhagic fever, 1975–1996. Adapted from WHO, 1997.

The risk of travellers to the tropics acquiring dengue fever is generally low. However, many travellers have acquired dengue during visits to epidemic areas.

**Prevention.** There is no vaccine for dengue fever; avoiding mosquito bites is the mainstay of prevention. Travellers to endemic areas should employ personal protection measures, including use of insect repellents, wearing clothes that reduce the amount of exposed skin and use of mosquito nets.

### Japanese encephalitis

Japanese encephalitis is a serious arboviral infection endemic in parts of Asia. Symptomatic illness is uncommon (1 in 300–1000 of those infected). For those who develop encephalitis, however, the case-fatality rate is 10–30%. Clinical illness is characterized by a non-specific prodrome following an incubation period of 6–16 days, progressing to meningismus, and symptoms and signs of encephalitis. Approximately 30% of encephalitis survivors have permanent neuropsychiatric sequelae. Diagnosis is by serology and treatment is supportive.

**Epidemiology.** Japanese encephalitis is endemic or epidemic throughout much of South-East Asia, the Indian subcontinent and East Asia (Figure 7.3). Distribution of the disease has been increasing, and cases have even been documented on the Australian mainland since 1998. The principal vector is *Culex tritaeniorhyncus*, a dusk-to-dawn biting mosquito, and typical high-risk regions have a combination of rice growing, pigs and birds. In some regions, sporadic cases occur year round; in other regions, seasonal epidemics occur, frequently after the rainy season (Table 7.1). Travellers at most risk are those travelling for extended periods to rural areas in which infection is endemic or where epidemic transmission is occurring.

**Prevention.** Vaccination is the principal means of prevention (see Chapter 5). An inactivated vaccine with a protective efficacy of about 95% is widely available. A primary course consists of three doses given over 1 month, with a single booster recommended every 3 years if the exposure risk continues. Generally, the vaccine is recommended for travellers spending an extended period (> 1 month) in endemic rural areas. Occasionally, the vaccine is recommended for those spending more than 1 year in urban areas within Japanese encephalitis endemic countries, or for short-term travellers in high-risk situations.

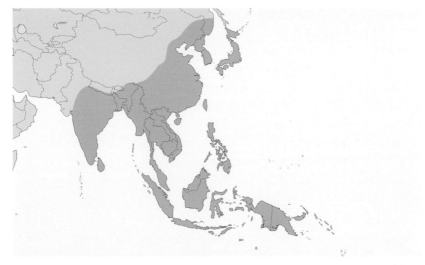

**Figure 7.3** Japanese encephalitis is endemic across much of South-East Asia and the Indian subcontinent (1970–1998). Adapted from Tsai *et al.*, 1999.

TABLE 7.1

**Geographical distribution and seasonal variations of Japanese encephalitis transmission**

| Country | Affected areas |
| --- | --- |
| Australia | Torres Strait Islands; occasional case in York Peninsula |
| Bangladesh | Probably widespread |
| Bhutan | Probably endemic in lowland areas, similar to Nepal |
| Brunei | Sporadic/endemic |
| Cambodia | Endemic/hyperendemic countrywide |
| China | All provinces except Tibet, Xinjiang and Qinghai. Hyperendemic in southern China |
| India | All states except Arunachal, Dadra, Daman, Diu, Gujarat, Himachal, Jammu, Kashmir, Lakshadweep, Meghalaya, Nagar Haveli, Orissa, Punjab, Rajasthan and Sikkim |
| Indonesia | Kalimantan, Bali, Nusa Tenggara, Sulawesi, Mollucas, Irian Jaya, Lombok |
| Japan | Rare cases on all islands, except Hokkaido |
| Korea | South Korea: sporadic/endemic with occasional outbreaks North Korea: no data |
| Laos | Endemic/hyperendemic countrywide |
| Malaysia | Sporadic/endemic in all states of Malaya, Sarawak and probably Sabah |
| Myanmar | Endemic/hyperendemic countrywide |
| Nepal | Hyperendemic in lowlands (Terai); occasional outbreaks in Kathmandu valley |
| Pakistan | Central delta areas |
| Papua New Guinea | Recent cases in North Fly District, Western Province |
| Philippines | Endemic in all islands |

| Transmission season | Comments |
| --- | --- |
| Probably year round | Rare cases reported from Australian mainland |
| Probably July–December | |
| Probably July–December | |
| Year round | |
| May–October | |
| North: May–September South: April–October | Rare cases in the New Territories of Hong Kong |
| Goa: May–October Tamil Nadu: October–January Karnataka: August–December (also April–June in Mandya District) Andra Pradesh: September–December North India: July–December | Regular outbreaks in West Bengal, Bihar, Karnataka, Tamil Nadu, Andhra Pradesh, Assam, Uttar Pradesh, Manipur and Goa |
| Probably year round. Peak risk: November–March, June–July | Rare cases reported among tourists to Bali |
| June–September Ryukyu islands: April–October | |
| July–October | |
| May–October | |
| Year round | Most cases from Penang, Perak, Selangor, Johore and Sarawak |
| May–October | Repeated outbreaks in Shan State and Chiang Mai Valley |
| July–December | Low risk for moderate- and high-altitude trekkers |
| June–January | Cases reported near Karachi |
| Year round in most areas, with peak risk April–January | Outbreaks in Nueva Ecija, Luzon and Manila |

TABLE 7.1 (continued)

| Country | Affected areas |
| --- | --- |
| Russia | Far eastern maritime areas south of Khabarousk |
| Singapore | Rare cases |
| Sri Lanka | Endemic in all but mountainous areas |
| Taiwan | Endemic/sporadic countrywide |
| Thailand | North: hyperendemic<br>South: sporadic/endemic |
| Vietnam | Endemic/hyperendemic countrywide |
| Western Pacific | Epidemics on Guam, Saipan (Northern Mariana Islands) |

## Other arthropod-borne infections

There are over 100 other known arboviruses that can infect humans, most of which are transmitted by mosquitoes. Most cause self-limiting acute febrile illness, though some can be life-threatening. With the ready availability of rapid travel by aircraft, the potential for spread of these viruses to previously non-endemic areas is great. This is illustrated by South Pacific outbreaks of Ross River fever and probably the recent outbreak of West Nile virus infection in New York city. Discussion of all these arboviral infections is beyond the scope of this book. However, their transmission usually occurs in a seasonal pattern, and travellers should be aware of ongoing outbreaks occurring in their destination countries. Filariasis and tick-borne encephalitis are discussed in Chapters 9 and 10, respectively.

| Transmission season | Comments |
| --- | --- |
| July–September | |
| Year round (April peak) | |
| October–January. Secondary peak: May–June | |
| April–October | Cases reported in and around Taipei |
| May–October | Regular outbreaks in Chiang Mai Valley. Sporadic cases in Bangkok suburbs |
| May–October | Highest rates in and near Hanoi |
| Possibly September–January | |

CHAPTER 8
# Food- and water-borne illnesses

Travellers may be exposed to a vast array of pathogens and chemicals via contaminated food and water (Table 8.1).

## Travellers' diarrhoea

**Epidemiology.** Travellers' diarrhoea (TD) is estimated to affect up to 10 million travellers every year. Destination is the greatest determinant of risk, with the highest risk destinations being the developing countries of Latin America, Africa, the Middle East and Asia (see Table 8.1 and Appendix A). Most travellers develop diarrhoea within 1 week of arrival at their destination, and attack rates of 20–50% in adults and up to 70% of children have been reported in some regions. Young children are more likely than adults to have a prolonged illness.

TD is acquired through the ingestion of faecally contaminated water or food. Consumption of raw (particularly unpeelable) fruit and vegetables, undercooked or raw meat and seafood, unpasteurized dairy products, ice and tap water is particularly risky. In general, eating food from street vendors has a higher risk than food in restaurants, which carries a higher risk than eating in private houses.

**Aetiology.** TD is caused by a wide variety of enteric pathogens. By far the most common pathogen worldwide is enterotoxigenic *Escherichia coli* (ETEC), which accounts for about 20–30% of all cases of TD. *Shigella*, *Salmonella* and *Campylobacter* are the most common causes of TD after ETEC, and their relative importance varies around the world. The number of organisms required to cause gastroenteritis depends on the organism and host factors. As few as 10 organisms can cause *Shigella* dysentery; 500 bacteria, *Campylobacter* gastroenteritis; $10^3$ organisms, salmonella, enterohaemorrhagic *E. coli* (EHEC) or enteroinvasive *E. coli* (EIEC) infections; and more than $10^8$ *E. coli* are required for ETEC diarrhoea.

Viruses, particularly rotavirus and Norwalk agent, have occasionally been implicated in TD. Many travellers have overemphasized the importance of enteric parasites, particularly *Giardia lamblia*. When specifically looked for, up to 6% of TD is caused by *G. lamblia* (Figure 8.1a), and a similar proportion by *Entamoeba histolytica*. *Cyclospora* has been recently recognized as an occasional cause of TD in many parts of the world (Figure 8.1b). *Cryptosporidium* may be a problem for the immunocompromised (Figure 8.1c). Approximately 20–50% of cases of TD have no documented infectious aetiology. This is due largely to the diagnostic limitations, though a small proportion of cases have non-infectious causes, such as drug side-effects or pre-existing gastrointestinal disorders.

**Clinical features.** In most cases, TD is a mild, self-limiting illness lasting 2–4 days, though 1% of sufferers will have prolonged diarrhoea ($\geq 1$ month). There may be other associated symptoms such as vomiting, anorexia, flatulence and abdominal pain. Fever does not occur in most cases, and is associated particularly with *Shigella*, *Salmonella* and *Campylobacter*. Dehydration can be life-threatening in children. Dysentery (blood and mucus) is associated particularly with *Shigella*, *Salmonella*, *Campylobacter*, *Yersinia* and EHEC.

**Prevention.** The ingestion of enteropathogens should be avoided. Travellers should be advised to avoid untreated water, consider water purification (boiling or halogenation) or drink only carbonated drinks (these have an antibacterial low pH). It is also important to avoid undercooked and reheated food, unpeelable fruit, ice cubes, unpasteurized milk and to adhere to strict personal hygiene. The simple adage is 'cook it, peel it or forget it'. Meticulous attention to such measures can decrease the risk of developing TD, though most travellers have difficulty adhering to these restrictions in practice.

*Water disinfection.* The most effective method of water sterilization is boiling. Less than 1 minute at 100°C is enough to kill all bacterial, protozoan and viral pathogens (a longer duration may be required at high altitude). The efficacy is not affected by the presence of sediment or the chemical composition of the water. Filtration is used widely and effectively removes bacteria, protozoal cysts and parasitic eggs, but not viruses. Most commercially available filters claim to remove bacteria and *Giardia*, and some incorporate halogen resins or activated charcoal to further aid disinfection.

TABLE 8.1

**Health hazards from water and food**

| Biology | Geographical distribution | Important sources | Incubation period |
| --- | --- | --- | --- |
| *Bacteria* | | | |
| *Campylobacter* spp. | Worldwide | Poultry, raw milk | 1–8 days |
| *Shigella* spp. | Worldwide | Egg salads, lettuce | 1–8 days |
| Non-typhoid salmonellae | Worldwide | Beef, poultry, eggs, dairy products | 6 hours–10 days |
| *Salmonella typhi* | Tropics | Water, shellfish, dairy products | 3 days–3 months |
| Enterotoxigenic *Escherichia coli* | Worldwide | Food and water | 6 hours–2 days |
| Enteropathogenic *Escherichia coli* | Mainly tropics | Food and water | 6 hours–2 days |
| Enterohaemorrhagic *Escherichia coli* | Worldwide | Beef, raw milk | 3–9 days |
| Enteroinvasive *Escherichia coli* | Tropics | Food and water | 1–8 days |
| *Vibrio cholerae* | Tropics | Shellfish | 4 hours–5 days |
| Non-cholera *Vibrio* spp. | Coastal areas | Seafood | 4–30 hours |
| *Yersinia enterocolitica* | Worldwide | Meat, milk | 3–7 days |
| *Aeromonas hydrophila* | Worldwide | Water | Unknown |
| *Pleisiomonas shigelloides* | Tropics | Water, shellfish | 1–2 days |
| *Staphylococcus aureus* | Worldwide | Ham, poultry, salads, pastries | 0.5–8 hours |
| *Bacillus cereus* | Worldwide | Fried rice, meats | 1–6 hours |
| *Clostridium perfringens* | Worldwide | Beef, poultry, gravy | 6–24 hours |
| *Clostridium botulinum* | Worldwide | Preserved food | 12 hours–days |
| *Listeria monocytogenes* | Worldwide | Meat, poultry, fish, dairy products | 3–70 days |

| Clinical features | Treatment |
| --- | --- |
| Diarrhoea, dysentery, abdominal pain | Supportive, macrolides, quinolones |
| Diarrhoea, dysentery | Supportive, quinolones |
| Diarrhoea, abdominal pain | Supportive, quinolones, third-generation cephalosporins |
| Enteric fever | Quinolones, third-generation cephalosporins |
| Diarrhoea | Supportive, quinolones, co-trimoxazole |
| Diarrhoea | Supportive, co-trimoxazole |
| Dysentery, haemolytic uraemic syndrome/ thrombotic thrombocytopaenic purpura | Supportive, role of antibiotics disputed |
| Diarrhoea, dysentery | Supportive, quinolones |
| Watery diarrhoea | Supportive, tetracycline |
| Diarrhoea, septicaemia (*Vibrio vulnificus*) | Supportive |
| Diarrhoea, abdominal pain | Supportive, quinolones, third-generation cephalosporins |
| Diarrhoea | Supportive, quinolones, co-trimoxazole |
| Diarrhoea | Supportive, quinolones, co-trimoxazole |
| Nausea, vomiting, diarrhoea | Supportive |
| Nausea and vomiting, or diarrhoea | Supportive |
| Diarrhoea, nausea | Supportive |
| Botulism | Supportive |
| Septicaemia, meningitis, diarrhoea | Ampicillin, aminoglycosides |

TABLE 8.1 (continued)

| Biology | Geographical distribution | Important sources | Incubation period |
|---------|---------------------------|-------------------|-------------------|
| *Viruses* | | | |
| Hepatitis A | Worldwide, particularly tropics | Food and water | 15–50 days |
| Hepatitis E | Worldwide, particularly tropics | Food and water | 15–64 days |
| Norwalk agent and Norwalk-like agents | Worldwide | Food, water, shellfish | 10–50 hours |
| Poliomyelitis | Africa, Asia | Food and water | 3–35 days |
| *Parasites* | | | |
| *Giardia lamblia* | Worldwide | Water and food | 3–25 days |
| *Entamoeba histolytica* | Worldwide | Food and water | Days to months |
| *Cryptosporidium parvum* | Worldwide | Food and water | 1–12 days |
| *Cyclospora cayatenensis* | Worldwide, mainly tropics | Food and water | 1–11 days |
| *Blastocystis hominis* | Worldwide | Food and water | Unknown |
| *Dientamoeba fragilis* | Worldwide | Water | Unknown |
| *Balantidium coli* | Worldwide | Food and water | Unknown |
| *Isospora belli* | Tropics, sub-tropics | Water | Approximately 1 week |
| Microsporidia | Worldwide | Water | Unknown |
| *Ascaris lumbricoides* | Worldwide | Vegetables | 4–8 weeks |
| *Trichuris trichiura* | Worldwide | Vegetables | Indefinite |
| *Capillaria philippinensis* | Mainly East and South-East Asia, Egypt | Fish | Unknown |
| *Angiostrongylus cantonensis* | South-East Asia, South Pacific | Snails, prawns, crabs, vegetables | 1–6 days |

| Clinical features | Treatment |
| --- | --- |
| Acute hepatitis | Supportive |
| Acute hepatitis | Supportive |
| Nausea, vomiting, diarrhoea | Supportive |
| Poliomyelitis | Supportive |
| Diarrhoea | Supportive, metronidazole, tinidazole |
| Dysentery, amoebic liver abscess | Supportive, metronidazole, tinidazole, diloxanide |
| Diarrhoea | Supportive, ?azithromycin |
| Diarrhoea | Supportive, co-trimoxazole |
| ?Diarrhoea | Supportive |
| Diarrhoea | Supportive, metronidazole |
| Diarrhoea, dysentery | Supportive, tetracycline, metronidazole |
| Diarrhoea | Co-trimoxazole |
| Diarrhoea | Metronidazole, albendazole |
| Asymptomatic, Löffler syndrome, nutritional deficiencies | Mebendazole, pyrantel, piperazine |
| Asymptomatic, dysentery, nutritional deficiencies | Mebendazole |
| Severe protein-losing enteropathy | Thiabendazole, albendazole, mebendazole |
| Eosinophilic meningitis | Supportive |

TABLE 8.1 (continued)

| Biology | Geographical distribution | Important sources | Incubation period |
|---|---|---|---|
| *Angiostrongylus costaricensis* | Central and South America | ?Food contaminated with slugs | |
| *Gnathostoma* spp. | South-East Asia, Japan, Latin America | Fish | |
| Anisakidae | Japan, The Netherlands, Scandinavia, Pacific Latin America | Saltwater fish, squid, octopus | Hours to days |
| *Fasciolopsis buski* | South-East Asia | Water caltrop, water chestnut | |
| *Fasciola hepatica* | Widespread in sheep- and cattle-raising areas | Watercress | Variable obstruction |
| *Clonorchis sinensis* | South-East Asia | Freshwater fish | Variable |
| *Paragonimus* spp. | East and South-East Asia, Africa, Americas | Freshwater crabs, crayfish | Variable |
| *Spirometra* spp. | East and South-East Asia | Fish, frogs, snakes | |
| *Diphyllobothrium latum* | Sub-Arctic, temperate and tropic zones | Fish | |
| *Taenia saginata* | Worldwide | Beef | |
| *Taenia solium* | Worldwide | Pork | Days to years |
| *Trichinella spiralis* | Worldwide | Pork and beef | 5–45 days |
| *Toxoplasma gondii* | Worldwide | Meat | 5–23 days |
| *Echinococcus granulosus* | Worldwide | Food and water | More than 1 year |

| Clinical features | Treatment |
|---|---|
| Abdominal pain | Removal, ?diethylcarbamazine + thiabendazole, ?metronidazole |
| Eosinophilic meningitis | Albendazole |
| Abdominal pain, cough | Removal |
| Diarrhoea, constipation, vomiting, anorexia | Praziquantel |
| Right upper quadrant pain, biliary | Bithionol |
| Abdominal pain, biliary obstruction | Praziquantel |
| Cough, haemoptysis, pleuritic chest pain | Praziquantel |
| Subcutaneous swellings, eye/CNS involvement | Removal |
| Asymptomatic, vitamin $B_{12}$ deficiency | Praziquantel, niclosamide |
| Intestinal disturbance | Niclosamide, praziquantel |
| Intestinal disturbance, neurocysticercosis | Niclosamide, praziquantel. Praziquantel + albendazole for cysticercosis |
| Asymptomatic, muscle pain, periorbital oedema, fever | Albendazole, thiabendazole |
| Asymptomatic, lymphadenopathy, cerebral toxoplasmosis in immunocompromised | Pyrimethamine + sulfadiazine + folinic acid |
| Symptoms associated with cyst locations | Removal, albendazole |

TABLE 8.1 (continued)

| Biology | Geographical distribution | Important sources | Incubation period |
|---|---|---|---|
| *Chemicals* | | | |
| Pufferfish poisoning | Japan, Atlantic coastal USA | Pufferfish | Under 3 hours |
| Ciguatera | South Pacific, Caribbean, Florida, Hawaii | Large predacious reef fish (e.g. barracuda) | 2–30 hours |
| Paralytic shellfish poisoning | Northern Pacific rim | Shellfish | 0.5–3 hours |
| Neurotoxic shellfish poisoning | Gulf and Atlantic coasts of Florida | Shellfish | Under 3 hours |
| Amnesic shellfish poisoning | Atlantic, Pacific and Indian Oceans | Shellfish | 0.5–36 hours |
| Diarrhoeic shellfish poisoning | Japan, Europe, South America | Shellfish | 0.5–30 hours |
| Scombroid fish poisoning | Worldwide | Tuna, mackerel, skipjack, bonito, albacore, bluefish | Minutes to hours |
| Mushroom poisoning | Worldwide | Mushrooms | Under 24 hours |
| Heavy metals | Worldwide | Acidic beverages | 5–15 minutes |
| Monosodium glutamate | Worldwide | Chinese food | Under 1 hour |

Halogenation is often more convenient than boiling, but is less effective particularly when the water has a high organic content, the temperature or halogen concentration is low, or the contact time is short. Iodine is more effective against protozoan cysts than chlorine, but both are active against viruses and bacteria. Organic material should be removed first by filtering and the manufacturers' instructions should be followed carefully to ensure a halogen concentration sufficient to kill pathogens, but not make the water unpalatable or unsafe. Lower concentrations or

| Clinical features | Treatment |
| --- | --- |
| Paraesthesiae, weakness, hypotension | Supportive |
| Nausea, vomiting, diarrhoea, abdominal pain | Supportive |
| Paraesthesiae | Supportive |
| Paraesthesiae, cerebellar and gastrointestinal symptoms | Supportive |
| Nausea, vomiting, headache, memory loss | Supportive |
| Nausea, vomiting, diarrhoea, abdominal pain | Supportive |
| Flushing, headache, dizziness | Antihistamine |
| Hallucinations, delirium, gastroenteritis, hepatic failure | Supportive |
| Nausea, vomiting, abdominal pain | Supportive |
| Burning sensation, headache, nausea, weakness, abdominal pain | Supportive |

temperatures need longer contact times (double the contact time for 4 ppm). Iodine is probably best avoided in those with uncontrolled thyroid disorders or iodine allergy, and pregnant women. Recommended halogen doses and contact times for various water temperatures are shown in Tables 8.2 and 8.3.

*Antimicrobial chemoprophylaxis* remains controversial. Although antimicrobials reduce the short-term rate of TD by up to 80–90% (Table 8.4), this must be balanced against the risk of adverse events and the

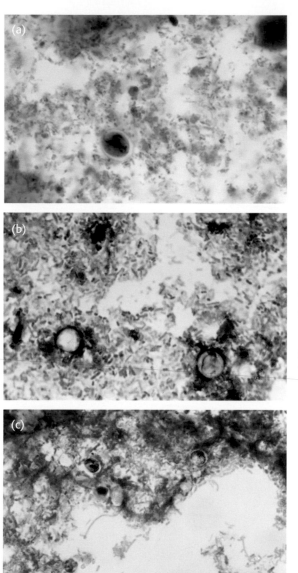

**Figure 8.1** Parasites causing travellers' diarrhoea: (a) *Giardia* spp., (b) *Cyclospora cayatenensis* and (c) *Cryptosporidium parvum* in different faecal samples.

potential for resistance to develop through widespread use. The most common adverse events include allergic reactions, antibiotic-associated colitis, vaginal candidiasis and photosensitivity reactions. Use of these agents can also lead to a false sense of security. Furthermore, their use poses a

TABLE 8.2

**Recommended halogen dose per litre of water for disinfection**

| Halogenation technique | Amount per litre for 4 ppm |
|---|---|
| Tetraglycine hydroperiodide tablets | ½ tablet |
| 2% iodine solution (tincture) | 0.2 ml, 5 drops |
| 10% povidone-iodine solution | 0.35 ml, 8 drops |
| Saturated iodine crystals in water | 14 ml |
| Saturated iodine crystals in alcohol | 0.1 ml for 5 ppm |
| Halazone tablets (mono-dichloraminobenzoic acid) | 2 tablets |
| Household bleach 5% (sodium hypochlorite) | 0.1 ml, 2 drops |

Adapted from Forgey WW, 1995

TABLE 8.3

**Chemical disinfection; recommended contact time for halogen at various water temperatures**

| Halogen concentration | Contact time at various water temperatures (minutes) | | |
|---|---|---|---|
| | 5°C | 15°C | 30°C |
| 4 ppm | 180 | 60 | 45 |
| 8 ppm | 60 | 30 | 15 |

Adapted from Forgey WW, 1995

difficulty when formulating a treatment plan should diarrhoea occur while a traveller is taking prophylactics. Given these reservations, the prophylactic use of antimicrobials is generally not recommended for travellers. However, they may be considered in certain restricted situations including travellers with underlying chronic illness that may be exacerbated by gastroenteritis and individuals making short trips, where illness would jeopardize the trip. Antibiotic chemoprophylaxis cannot be recommended for children unless

TABLE 8.4

**Drugs for prophylaxis of travellers' diarrhoea**

| Agent | Adult dosage |
| --- | --- |
| Norfloxacin | 400 mg daily |
| Ciprofloxacin | 500 mg daily |
| Ofloxacin | 300 mg daily |
| Levofloxacin | 400 mg daily |
| Co-trimoxazole | 160/800 mg daily |
| Bismuth subsalicylate | 2 tablets with meals at night |

there is an underlying medical risk factor that should be considered, and the period of risk is short.

**Vaccines** directed against agents implicated in TD are being evaluated currently. None is likely to be widely available in the near future.

*ETEC.* Trials of an inactivated whole-cell oral vaccine against ETEC have demonstrated safety and immunogenicity in children and adults, and 50% protective efficacy against ETEC in adults.

*Shigella.* Trials of *Shigella* protein–polysaccharide conjugate vaccines in adults and children have shown it to be safe and immunogenic. Early efficacy data suggest that these vaccines afford more than 70% protection in adults, though the duration of protection is not yet clear. Attenuated live *Shigella* vaccines have been shown to be protective in challenge studies and are now in trials.

*Campylobacter.* An oral killed whole-cell vaccine against *Campylobacter jejuni* has demonstrated immunogenicity and safety in animal models and is currently in clinical trials. Subunit vaccines are in the early stages of development in animal models.

*Rotavirus.* A vaccine was licensed in the USA for routine use in infants in 1998 after trials demonstrated immunogenicity, safety and efficacy. Immunization was subsequently found to be associated with intussusception in infants and the vaccine was withdrawn by the manufacturer in October 1999.

**Treatment.** TD is generally a self-limiting illness, with acute complications or chronic symptoms developing in a minority. The mainstay of treatment is fluid and electrolyte replacement; spread is prevented by careful handwashing. The combination of an antimicrobial and an antimotility agent is recommended in adults to shorten the duration of symptoms. Quinolones are currently the most effective agents because of the increasing resistance to ampicillin and doxycycline. However, quinolone resistance in salmonellae and *Campylobacter* spp. has become an increasing problem in South-East Asia. Azithromycin might be considered for quinolone-resistant *Campylobacter* spp. Loperamide is a useful adjunct to rehydration and antimicrobial therapy. It should be noted, however, that antimotility agents are contraindicated in children AND when the diarrhoea is bloody (dysentery). Although food stimulates the gastrocolic reflex and can cause abdominal discomfort, eating should be encouraged if tolerable as maintenance of adequate nutrition can be an important therapeutic measure.

For moderate to severe diarrhoea (three or more loose motions per day), single-dose antimicrobial therapy plus loperamide is recommended. If symptoms do not improve after 12 hours, standard dosing should be continued for 3 full days. For severe diarrhoea with incapacitating symptoms, fever or bloody motions, an antimicrobial agent should be administered at a standard dose for 3 days. Single doses may be insufficient to eradicate salmonella infection (Table 8.5).

*In children*, TD may be severe and lead to serious dehydration, so oral rehydration is the mainstay of treatment. Parents travelling to high-risk areas with young children should carry commercially available electrolyte mixtures; homemade recipes are often prepared incorrectly and may lead to hypernatraemia.

For specific treatment, antibiotics may limit the duration of the illness and should be used with oral rehydration. For short-treatment courses, quinolones are most useful. Fears about joint toxicity in children, based on data from animal studies, do not seem to have been justified clinically, and recent studies suggest that short courses of quinolones are acceptable in children. Antimotility agents should be avoided.

**Persistent symptoms.** Of those with TD, 3% suffer for more than 14 days and 1–2% for more than 30 days. By this stage, first-line therapy, usually

TABLE 8.5

**Drugs for the treatment of travellers' diarrhoea**

| Drug | Doses | |
|------|-------|-|
| | Adults | Children |
| Norfloxacin | 800 mg once **OR** 400 mg twice daily for 3 days | 800 mg once **OR** 400 mg twice daily for 3 days |
| Ciprofloxacin | 1000 mg once **OR** 500 mg twice daily for 3 days | 5–10 mg/kg/dose twice daily for 3 days (max 750 mg) |
| Co-trimoxazole | 320/1600 mg once **OR** 160/800 mg twice daily for 3 days | 5/25 mg/kg twice daily for 3 days |
| Metronidazole | 2 g daily as a single dose for 3 days | 7.5 mg/kg per dose three times daily for 3 days (maximum 800 mg) |
| Tinidazole | 2 g daily as a single dose for 3 days | 50 mg/kg single dose for 3 days |
| Loperamide | 4 mg initially, then 2 mg after each loose motion (maximum 16 mg/day) | Not recommended |

with a quinolone, has failed and an alternative diagnosis should be suspected. At this time (7–10 days), stool cultures should be examined, if possible, and empirical therapy with metronidazole or tinidazole administered for 7 days for suspected *Giardia* or *Entamoeba*. *Isospora* and *Cyclospora* have recently been implicated as common causes of prolonged (> 3 weeks) diarrhoea, and are effectively treated with co-trimoxazole (10-day course). Cryptosporidium is usually self-limiting, except in the immunocompromised, and specific therapy is not indicated.

**Cholera**

Cholera is an acute intestinal infection caused by toxigenic strains of *Vibrio cholerae* O1 or O139. Infection is generally waterborne, but may be associated with shellfish or other contaminated food.

**Epidemiology.** Cholera occurs widely throughout the tropics. Areas with highest risk include India, South-East Asia, Africa, the Middle East, Southern Europe, Oceania, South America (Peru) and the Gulf of Mexico. Most outbreaks occur in the warmer months and are associated with seafood. The risk for travellers is very low (probably < 1:500 000).

**Clinical features.** Infection with *Vibrio cholerae* is often asymptomatic. However, the most common clinical disease is painless, watery diarrhoea without fever occurring from a few hours to a few days after exposure. In some people, stools may be of high volume and contain some mucus ('rice-water' stool). In the most severe cases (5%), dehydration may occur within 12 hours of onset of diarrhoea, resulting in acidosis, hypoglycaemia, hypovolaemia, coma and convulsions.

**Prevention.** The general precautions for the prevention of TD apply to cholera.

**Vaccines.** A killed whole-cell oral vaccine is no longer widely available as it provided limited personal protection (50%) and was unable to control outbreaks. However, an oral live attenuated vaccine has been shown to be safe, immunogenic and protective. The risk of cholera is very low for travellers, but this vaccine may be useful for those in areas that have outbreaks, particularly aid workers.

**Treatment.** Oral rehydration with a balanced glucose/electrolyte solution is the mainstay of treatment and is life-saving in severe cases. Intravenous rehydration may be necessary in those unable to take oral or nasogastric fluids. Antibiotics reduce the duration of diarrhoea and can be used in all but the mildest cases. Tetracycline, doxycycline, co-trimoxazole, quinolones and erythromycin are often effective. Resistance to tetracyclines is reported and some serotypes are inherently resistant to co-trimoxazole.

## Typhoid

Typhoid fever is an acute febrile illness caused by *Salmonella typhi*. Typhoid is associated with faecally contaminated food and drink. This general clinical syndrome is often referred to as enteric fever and may be caused by other

79

bacteria, including *Salmonella paratyphi*, *Yersinia enterocolitica* and *Campylobacter fetus*.

**Epidemiology.** *Salmonella typhi* is endemic in Africa, Asia, Central and South America, the Caribbean and some areas in Eastern Europe, and is found only in humans (unlike other salmonellae). Risk is generally low, but can be as high as 1:3000 for travellers to the Indian subcontinent, north and west Africa, and parts of South America.

**Clinical features.** The incubation period for typhoid fever is usually 1–2 weeks, but symptoms have been documented from a few days to 2 months after infection. Onset is characterized by fever, headache, malaise and anorexia. Gastrointestinal symptoms may not be prominent initially. Abdominal pain, hepatosplenomegaly and rose spots can occur and may be accompanied by constipation. Diarrhoea may occur in the second week. Excretion of *S. typhi* continues for months after infection and, in 1%, may continue for a year.

**Prevention.** The general precautions to avoid TD apply to the prevention of typhoid.

**Vaccines.** Several typhoid vaccines have been available in recent years. No vaccine approaches 100% efficacy.

**Treatment.** Multidrug-resistant *S. typhi* has become increasingly common in recent years, and empirical treatment with chloramphenicol, ampicillin or co-trimoxazole may fail. Fluoroquinolones are currently most convenient for oral therapy. In young children and for intravenous therapy, a third-generation cephalosporin or ciprofloxacin are the most commonly used agents when resistant strains are possible. Public health measures are important in limiting spread.

### Poliomyelitis

Poliomyelitis is an acute viral gastrointestinal tract infection that occasionally involves the central nervous system. The majority of infections are asymptomatic, but a proportion are associated with neurological features, including flaccid paralysis and respiratory failure. Poliomyelitis is acquired by faecal–oral transmission, and has been particularly common in areas of poor hygiene and sanitation. The incidence of poliomyelitis has fallen dramatically with the widespread use of polio vaccines, and improved sanitation and hygiene. It is hoped that the disease will soon be completely eradicated, as it is in North and South America, but transmission continues in parts of Africa, Asia, the Middle East and Eastern Europe. Travellers to countries with ongoing transmission should be fully immunized.

## Hepatitis A and E

Hepatitis A and E are covered in Chapter 11.

## Angiostrongyliasis

Human infection with the rat lungworm, *Angiostrongylus cantonensis*, is associated with meningitis and increased numbers of eosinophils in the cerebrospinal fluid and peripheral blood (eosinophilic meningitis). Generally, infection is mild and self-limiting (there is no specific therapy), but fatalities have been occasionally documented, primarily in the South Pacific and South-East Asia. Transmission occurs through the ingestion of raw or undercooked snails, prawns or crabs, or other foods exposed to snails or slugs (both intermediate hosts of the worm), such as leafy vegetables. *A. cantonensis* infection should be considered in people with eosinophilic meningitis who have recently visited endemic areas.

Human infection with *Angiostrongylus costaricensis* is characterized by abdominal pain, vomiting, eosinophilia and a right lower quadrant mass. Most cases have come from Central and South America, and transmission to humans probably occurs in a similar manner to *A. cantonensis*.

## Fish and shellfish poisoning syndromes

Fish and shellfish poisoning syndromes occur as a consequence of consuming seafood contaminated with toxins produced by certain dinoflagellates/algae (plankton). Six main syndromes are recognized.

**Ciguatera fish poisoning** is the most widely recognized, and illness results from eating large, predacious reef fish, such as barracuda, snapper, amberjack and groper. Ciguatera fish poisoning is particularly common in

81

parts of the tropical South Pacific and Caribbean. Typically, gastrointestinal symptoms begin 6 hours after consumption of fish (which tastes and appears normal), followed by neurological symptoms such as paraesthesiae, itching, myalgias and temperature reversal. Occasionally, serious complications do occur, but the condition is usually self-limiting.

**Paralytic shellfish poisoning** follows consumption of shellfish harvested from affected areas, particularly around the USA (Alaska, Pacific north-west coast and coastal New England), the Philippines and the North Sea. Neurological symptoms predominate.

**Neurotoxic shellfish poisoning** occurs following consumption of shellfish harvested from the Gulf of Mexico, west coast of Florida and New Zealand. Both neurological and gastrointestinal symptoms occur within minutes to hours of ingestion. Eye irritation can occur following aerosolization of toxin by wave action.

**Diarrhoetic shellfish poisoning** has had outbreaks in Japan, Europe, New Zealand, Canada and South America. Diarrhoea (often severe), nausea and vomiting occur within 2 hours of ingestion, and resolve within about a day.

**Amnesic shellfish poisoning** has occurred in outbreaks in the Atlantic provinces of Canada and coastal USA. Gastrointestinal followed by neurological symptoms predominate. Short-term memory deficits are common, and may persist for months.

*Pfiesteria*-**associated syndrome** following water exposure along the coast and from major rivers has been seen in the mid-Atlantic states of the USA, particularly Maryland and North Carolina. Eye, skin and respiratory tract irritation, and neurological symptoms have been described as part of the syndrome.

**Prevention** of fish and shellfish poisoning involves avoidance of seafood harvested from high-risk areas. In all cases, treatment is supportive only.

CHAPTER 9
# Other parasitic diseases

The parasitic infections discussed in this chapter are of varying, often low, risk to travellers. Most are characterized by chronic illness, often with potentially serious sequelae.

## Schistosomiasis (bilharzia)

Schistosomiasis is caused by blood flukes (schistosomes), and is now recognized as an important travellers' disease. Five species of schistosomes can cause human disease, and their geographical distribution and clinical features vary. *Schistosoma mansoni*, *Schistosoma haematobium* and *Schistosoma intercalatum* are found mainly in Africa, though other foci exist in South and Central America, the Middle East and India (Figure 9.1). *Schistosoma japonicum* and *Schistosoma mekongi* are found in foci throughout South-East Asia. Infection is acquired through contact with freshwater lakes and rivers containing larval forms of the parasite (cercariae;

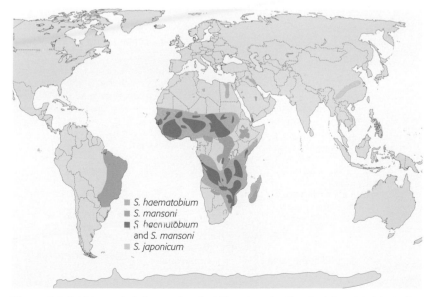

S. haematobium
S. mansoni
S. haematobium
and S. mansoni
S. japonicum

**Figure 9.1** Schistosomiasis is prevalent in Africa, though other foci do exist. Adapted from WHO website, 2000.

see Figure 9.2). Cercariae emerge from a snail intermediate host and are able to penetrate intact skin. Thereafter, the larvae enter the bloodstream and migrate to various organs. Eventually, the mature adult flukes migrate to abdominal veins; *S. haematobium* resides in the vesical plexus of the bladder, while the other species usually remain in the mesenteric veins. Eggs are deposited in the lumen of the bladder or bowel, but occasionally lodge in other organs such as the central nervous system.

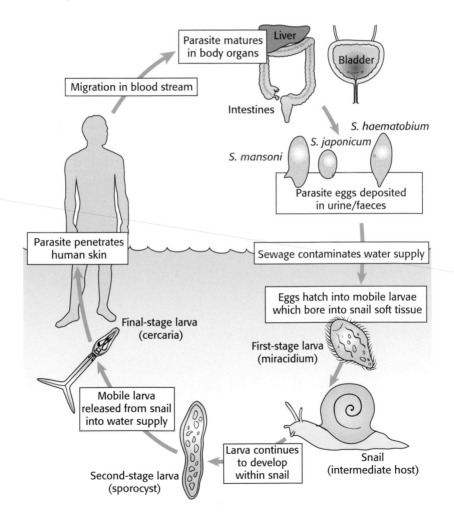

**Figure 9.2** The life cycle of a schistosome.

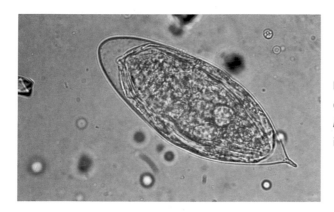

**Figure 9.3** Ova of *Schistosoma haematobium* seen in a urine sample.

The number of reported cases in travellers has increased steadily in recent years. The major risk areas include Lake Malawi, the Nile River valley and Lake Victoria. Lake Malawi has received particular attention and, contrary to local advice, schistosomes are present throughout the lake. Travellers should avoid swimming or wading in freshwater bodies in endemic areas. Travellers who may have been exposed to schistosomes should be screened after their travels, even if asymptomatic.

**Clinical features** can occur at several stages in the life cycle of the fluke. Within 24 hours of exposure, a pruritic papular rash may appear at the site of cercariae penetration (swimmers' itch). The next clinical syndrome, known as Katayama fever, occurs 4–8 weeks later and coincides with the start of oviposition. Features include fever, chills, headache, splenomegaly, hepatomegaly, lymphadenopathy and eosinophilia. Most symptoms disappear within days or weeks, but occasionally acute schistosomiasis can be fatal, particularly when caused by *S. japonicum*. In general, the chronic complications of schistosomiasis are the most important. Chronic schistosomiasis can occur years after exposure and is a result of the host response to *Schistosoma* ova (Figure 9.3). Complications include obstructive uropathy, bladder cancer, hepatic fibrosis and portal hypertension.

**Diagnosis.** The diagnosis of schistosomiasis relies on the detection of ova in faeces and/or urine (ideally collected between 10.00 and 14.00 hours), or in rectal biopsy specimens. Serology can be a useful screening test for travellers who normally reside in areas not endemic for schistosomiasis. High titres in such travellers are an indication for treatment. Schistosomiasis is safely and effectively treated with oral praziquantel.

## Chagas' disease

Chagas' disease is a serious disease caused by the protozoan *Trypanosoma cruzi*, which is endemic in regions of South and Central America, and Brazil in particular (Figure 9.4). Travellers to populated poor rural areas in Brazil are at most risk. Transmission between humans is via triatomine bugs found in the crevices of dirt walls of houses. Transmission can also occur through blood transfusion. *T. cruzi* resides in the blood and macrophages in various organs, including the heart and gastrointestinal tract. Chronic, irreversible, life-threatening sequelae may occur many years after asymptomatic infection, and sequelae include dilated cardiomyopathy, megaoesophagus and megacolon. Treatment is limited and often ineffective, particularly for chronic disease.

**Prevention.** Bug bites should be avoided, as should sleeping in adobe buildings in endemic areas. Blood transfusions while in endemic areas are inadvisable.

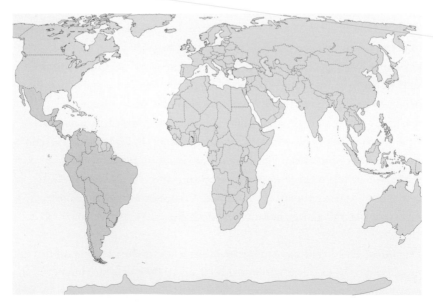

**Figure 9.4** The geographical distribution of Chagas' disease. Adapted from WHO, 1996.

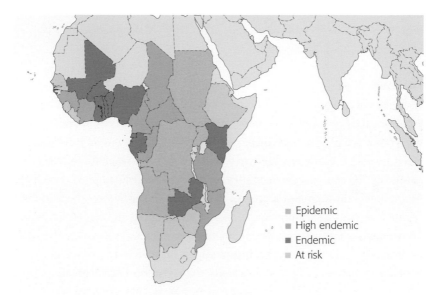

Epidemic
High endemic
Endemic
At risk

**Figure 9.5** Distribution of African trypanosomiasis. Adapted from WHO, 1997.

**African trypanosomiasis (sleeping sickness)** is endemic throughout much
of sub-Saharan Africa (Figure 9.5), and its prevalence is increasing in
many countries. The disease is caused by two *Trypanosoma* sub-species,
*Trypanosoma brucei gambiense* and *Trypanosoma brucei rhodesiense*,
which are transmitted by tsetse fly bites. Each subspecies causes a distinct
epidemiological disease. Humans are the primary reservoir of west African
trypanosomiasis, caused by *T. brucei gambiense*, and transmission occurs
mainly in wooded areas beside rivers. East African trypanosomiasis is caused
by *T. brucei rhodesiense*, and antelope and cattle are the primary reservoirs.
Transmission occurs mainly in savannah and woodland areas. East and west
African trypanosomiasis both have an early stage characterized by fever,
musculoskeletal pain, headache, lymphadenopathy and rash, followed by
more pronounced systemic manifestations. The central nervous system is
involved in advanced stages, and behaviour and sleep patterns are altered.
Untreated, it is fatal.

Only rarely is African trypanosomiasis seen in travellers, but it has been
acquired by visitors to east African game parks. Travellers visiting remote
rural areas or taking wildlife safaris are at most risk, while travellers to
urban areas only are not at risk. Arms and legs should be covered and insect

87

repellents used when visiting endemic areas, and car windows should be kept closed while travelling.

## Filariasis

Filariasis encompasses several diseases caused by roundworms. All are transmitted by mosquitoes or other flies, cause peripheral eosinophilia, and involve the lymphatics and connective tissues. Although rare in travellers, three are seen occasionally and are worth a mention. Lymphatic filariasis is caused by *Wuchereria bancrofti*, *Brugia malayi* and *Brugia timori*, which are found in foci throughout the tropics (Figure 9.6). Adult worms dwell in the lymphatics, causing lymphangitis, lymphadenitis and lymphatic obstruction. Elephantiasis describes the resulting permanent skin and soft-tissue changes. As infection is transmitted by mosquito bites, prevention is directed at avoidance of bites. In the Pacific Islands, the mosquito vectors are most active during the day, while in other endemic areas, they are most active at night.

## Onchocerciasis (river blindness)

Onchocerciasis is caused by *Onchocerca volvulus* and is endemic in equatorial Africa (particularly west Africa), small foci in Yemen, northern

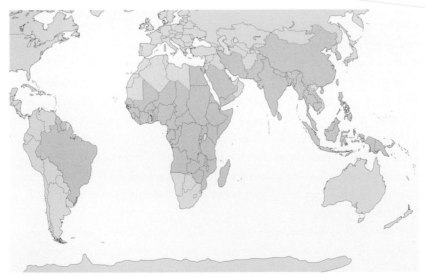

**Figure 9.6** Lymphatic filariasis is prevalent in foci throughout the tropics.

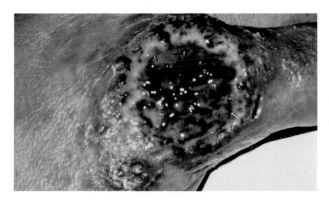

**Figure 9.7**
Cutaneous leishmaniasis on a traveller returning from South America.

South America and Central America. Dermatitis is the major clinical manifestation, but eye involvement leading to blindness is the most serious. Black flies that breed in fast-flowing rivers and streams transmit the infection.

## Loiasis

*Loa loa* is transmitted by day-biting deer flies, and is found in rainforests of west and central Africa. Subcutaneous swellings are the major clinical feature.

## Leishmaniasis

*Leishmania*, which is transmitted by the bite of infected phlebotomine sandflies, cause leishmaniasis. Three major clinical syndromes reflect the species or subspecies of infecting parasite, the host immune status and the location of the infected macrophages:

- visceral leishmaniasis is a chronic systemic illness characterized by fever, chills, weight loss and hepatosplenomegaly, which has a high mortality if untreated. HIV-infected individuals are at increased risk
- cutaneous leishmaniasis has hallmark chronic, painless skin ulcers (Figure 9.7)
- mucocutaneous leishmaniasis arises as a complication when some New World species of *Leishmania* involve mucosal surfaces.

Leishmaniasis is uncommon in travellers, but the diagnosis should be considered when faced with ulcerating skin lesions following travel to an endemic area. Diagnosis usually relies on demonstration of the parasite in affected tissue. The sandfly vectors are weak fliers and feed at night, so wearing clothing that covers arms and legs at night and sleeping upstairs can help prevent bites.

## Intestinal roundworms

Travellers may be exposed to intestinal roundworms such as *Ascaris lumbricoides*, whipworm (*Trichuris trichuria*), hookworms and *Strongyloides stercoralis*, particularly while travelling in the tropics. Long-term travellers in regions endemic for these parasites should be screened after their travels.

## Cutaneous larva migrans

This dermatitis, or 'creeping eruption', is caused by the dog or cat hookworms *Ancylostoma braziliense* or *Ancylostoma caninum*. Larvae penetrate the skin, particularly of the feet, and migrate intracutaneously producing a serpiginous track. Because these parasites are maladapted to humans, further maturation does not occur and invasion of deeper tissues is rare. Those at greatest risk for cutaneous larva migrans are people in contact with damp sandy soil contaminated with dog or cat faeces, particularly those without footwear.

## Myiasis

Myiasis refers to the invasion of tissue by fly larvae (maggots). Several flies are capable of causing human myiasis, though two are particularly relevant to travellers. Both cause boil-like skin lesions that can be mistaken for bacterial abscesses. The human botfly (*Dermatobia hominis*) is endemic in lowland forests of Central America and tropical South America. Female flies cement their eggs to the abdomen of captured mosquitoes. When the carrier mosquito lands on a mammal, the larvae hatch and penetrate into the mammal's subcutaneous tissue, where they mature to adult flies. The Tumbu fly (*Cordylobia anthropophagia*) exists throughout sub-Saharan Africa. Female flies lay eggs on soil or clothing, and larvae invade subcutaneous tissue after hatching, where they mature to adults.

Prevention of mosquito bites will help prevent botfly infestation. In Tumbu fly-endemic areas, clothing and towels left outside to dry should be ironed before use. When discovered, larvae of both species can be very

difficult to remove. The best technique involves applying a substance –
petroleum jelly, chewing gum and pork fat have all been used successfully –
to the lesion to asphyxiate the larvae.

## Tungiasis

The flea *Tunga penetrans* (jigger) is found in tropical Africa, Madagascar,
Central America, tropical South America and the Caribbean. The female
flea penetrates soft skin around the toes, where she feeds and distends
enormously, eventually attaining the size of a pea. After 2–3 weeks, female
fleas discharge their eggs and eventually die. Clinical manifestations result
from inflammation and secondary infection. Wearing shoes is the most
effective preventative measure.

CHAPTER 10
# Diseases transmitted by ticks, lice, mites and fleas

Ticks, lice, mites and fleas are vectors of a number of infections, some of which are encountered only rarely by travellers. In general, avoiding these vectors and their bites is the primary, if not only, preventative measure. Some vaccines are available, but only tick-borne encephalitis vaccine has been administered to travellers on a regular basis.

## Rickettsial infections
Rickettsia infections are usually separated into two groups, typhus and spotted fevers. Both groups share many features, including transmission by arthropods, treatment with doxycycline and the characteristic clinical triad of headache, fever and rash.

**Typhus.** There are three diseases within this group caused by different microorganisms.

*Epidemic (louse-borne) typhus* is caused by *Rickettsia prowazekii* and is characterized by the acute onset of headache, fever, general aches and pains, followed by a macular eruption. The incubation period is 1–2 weeks. The disease can be severe, with case-fatality rates of 10–40% if untreated. In compromised hosts, recrudescence can occur years after the primary attack (Brill–Zinsser disease). Humans are the reservoir, and transmission is via the body louse *Pediculus humanus*. Epidemic typhus occurs mainly when conditions favour lice proliferation, such as during cold weather and during war or natural disasters. Endemic foci exist in the mountainous regions of Central and South America, in east Africa and in many areas of Asia. Occasionally, cases linked to flying squirrels, which serve as a reservoir, occur in the USA, particularly the East Coast states. Epidemic typhus is uncommon in travellers, and conditions that favour transmission should be avoided.

*Murine (endemic) typhus* is caused by *Rickettsia typhi*, and has a clinical course that resembles, but is less severe than, epidemic typhus. The case-fatality rate is less than 1%. Rats, mice and other mammals serve as reservoirs, and transmission to humans is through infected rat-flea bites. Murine typhus occurs worldwide, and is particularly common in areas where humans occupy rat- and mice-infested buildings. Many cases have been reported in travellers, particularly those returning from South-East Asia. Travellers should avoid buildings infested with rats and mice.

*Scrub typhus* is caused by *Orientia* (formerly *Rickettsia*) *tsutsugamushi*, and has a clinical picture of fever, headache, lymphadenopathy and conjunctival infection, followed by a maculopapular eruption. The incubation period is 6–21 days. Untreated, the case-fatality rate is 1–60%, depending on geographical area, bacterial strain and age. Transmission occurs through the bite of infected larval mites (chiggers) of the genus *Leptotrombidium*, and an eschar is often found at the attachment site. Mites infest sharply demarcated areas in scrub terrain between forest and clearings within parts of Asia (Figure 10.1). When traversing such areas, humans

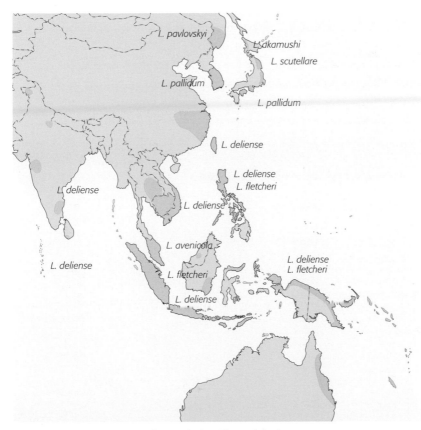

**Figure 10.1** Areas in Asia and Australasia with scrub typhus.

become accidental hosts. Protective clothing (particularly covering the lower extremities) should be worn and insect repellent applied while walking through endemic areas.

**Spotted fevers** encompass a range of diseases characterized by acute febrile illnesses with generalized rashes (Table 10.1). The rash is usually maculopapular, except in the case of rickettsialpox, which produces a widespread vesicular rash that can be confused with chickenpox. All, except Rocky Mountain spotted fever, are associated with the presence of an eschar.

### Tick-borne encephalitis

Tick-borne encephalitis (TBE) is the major tick-borne viral infection of relevance to travellers. It is caused by two viral subtypes, Central European and Far Eastern (Russian spring-summer encephalitis). Most infected individuals are either asymptomatic or have a mild 'flu-like' illness. However, a sizeable minority develop meningeal and/or encephalitic syndromes, occasionally associated with focal neurological deficits. The case-fatality rate is high (20% for the Far-Eastern type) and as many as half of survivors have neuropsychiatric sequelae. TBE circulates in small

TABLE 10.1

**Spotted fever group of rickettsial diseases**

| Disease | Organism | Distribution | Vector | Vertebrate hosts |
|---------|----------|--------------|--------|------------------|
| Rocky Mountain spotted fever | *Rickettsia rickettsii* | North, Central and South America | Tick | Rodents, dogs |
| Boutoneuse fever | *Rickettsia conori* | Mediterranean, Africa, India | Tick | Rodents, dogs |
| Queensland tick typhus | *Rickettsia australis* | Australia | Tick | Rodents, marsupials |
| North Asian tick typhus | *Rickettsia sibirica* | Siberia, Mongolia | Tick | Rodents |
| Rickettsialpox | *Rickettsia akari* | North America, Russia, South Africa, Korea | Mite | Mouse |

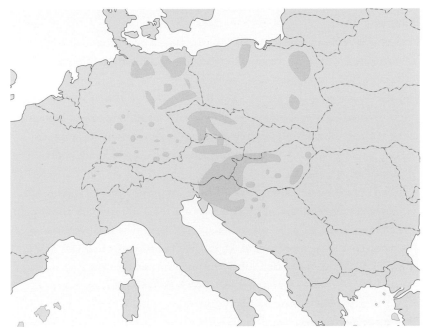

**Figure 10.2** Parts of Eastern Europe with tick-borne encephalitis.

mammals, particularly rodents, and is transmitted to humans by infected
ticks or by drinking milk from infected cows, sheep or goats. The infection is
distributed throughout Eastern Europe and parts of East Asia (Figure 10.2).
Seasonal epidemics occur in spring and early summer in Russia, and from
late spring to early autumn in Europe.

Campers and hikers who walk through forests in affected areas during
the epidemic season are particularly at risk, but generally the risk to
travellers is very low. Tick-infested areas should be avoided, insect repellents
used and protective clothing worn.

**Inactivated TBE vaccine**, which is safe, effective and protects against
both serotypes, is available in Europe, but difficult to obtain elsewhere.
Administered as three doses given at 0, 1–3 and 9–12 months, the
protection rate is more than 98% and lasts for 3–5 years. Several other rapid
vaccination schedules have shown similar efficacy. Side-effects are infrequent
and usually relate to reactions at the injection site. Egg allergy is a relative
contraindication to administration.

## Relapsing fever

Relapsing fever is an acute systemic disease caused by various spirochaetes of the genus *Borrelia*. There are two types of infection with different causative agents and modes of transmission.

- Louse-borne relapsing fever is caused by *Borrelia recurrentis* and is transmitted between humans by body lice, *Pediculus humanus*. Humans are the only host for this species. It is restricted to certain locations in Asia, and highland areas of east and central Africa and South America, particularly the Andes.
- Tick-borne relapsing fever is caused by many other *Borrelia* species and is transmitted to humans by soft ticks (*Ornithodoros* spp.). Reservoirs include chipmunks, squirrels, rabbits, rats, mice, owls and even lizards. It is endemic throughout tropical Africa, and occasionally in north Africa, the Middle East, the Indian subcontinent and South America. Cases have also been reported in parts of south-western North America, where rodents carry the disease into human areas.

Both types share clinical features, in particular recurrent febrile episodes and petechial rash. Mortality is as high as 40% in louse-borne relapsing fever and 5% for the tick-borne disease.

Reports of travellers with relapsing fever are rare and prevention relies on personal protection against louse infestation and tick bites. Tetracycline is the treatment of choice.

## Lyme disease

Lyme disease is a spirochaetal infection caused by *Borrelia burgdorferi* in North America, and *B. burgdorferi*, *Borrelia garinii*, *Borrelia afzelii* and others elsewhere. Transmission occurs through infected *Ixodes* tick bites. Clinical manifestations have different stages, and include fever, erythema migrans, neurological symptoms and arthritis. Travellers who visit forested regions within endemic areas of North America (particularly the north-east, north-central and coastal Pacific regions; Figure 10.3), and temperate forested regions of Europe and Asia are at most risk. Lyme disease has not yet been convincingly demonstrated in Australia. Travellers should use insect repellents and avoid tick bites. A vaccine against North American Lyme disease agents is available, but is unlikely to be highly effective in other regions.

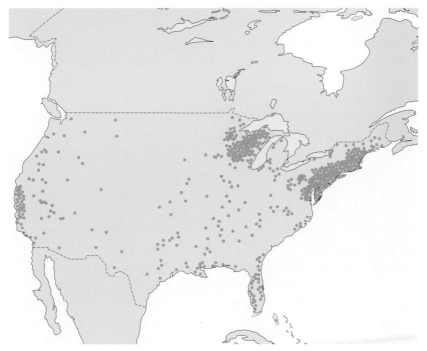

**Figure 10.3** Prevalence of Lyme disease in the USA, 1998.

## Plague

Plague is a zoonosis transmitted by infected rodent fleas. The fleas bite humans, and human-to-human transmission can occur through droplet spread from patients with pneumonic plague. Plague remains endemic in many parts of Africa, North and South America, and Asia. However, the disease is very rare in travellers.

A vaccine is available, but is generally only recommended for people working in plague-enzootic areas, those working with patients with plague and laboratory personnel working with *Yersinia pestis.*

CHAPTER 11

# Miscellaneous infectious diseases

## Meningococcal disease

Although meningococcal disease is rare amongst travellers, vaccinations are recommended for those visiting epidemic areas. Current vaccines produce short-lived immunity for serogroups A, C, Y and W135 disease. New vaccines that offer the possibility of long-lasting protection are under development.

**Epidemiology.** Meningococci are carried asymptomatically in the nasopharynx of 10% of healthy adults at any time. Despite such high carriage rates, meningococcal disease is very uncommon. The incidence of invasive disease caused by *Neisseria meningitidis* ranges from less than 1 in 100 000 in many areas of the USA to more than 12 in 100 000 in New Zealand. However, during the dry season in an epidemic year in some parts of sub-Saharan Africa, the incidence can be as high as 1000 in 100 000 in discrete communities. This area of Africa, extending from Senegal to Ethiopia, has become known as the meningitis belt of Africa (Figure 11.1). Recent epidemics have extended south and have been associated particularly with refugee camps. This area extends through the Middle East (Saudi Arabia) into Asia (Nepal, India, China and Mongolia), though epidemics outside Africa have not been reported in recent years. Some authorities still require evidence of vaccination.

Meningococcal disease is associated with young age (the greatest risk is 6–24 months), winter/dry season, crowded conditions and tobacco smoking. Complement deficiencies (C3 and C5–9), hypogammaglobulinaemia and hyposplenism also increase the risk of disease.

Serogroups A, B, C, Y and W135 commonly cause invasive disease. Each serogroup is defined by the biochemical structure of its polysaccharide capsule. In industrialized countries, serogroup B meningococci are responsible for two-thirds of cases of invasive disease. Serogroup C meningococci account for the majority of remaining cases, though serogroup Y disease has become more common in the United States in recent years.

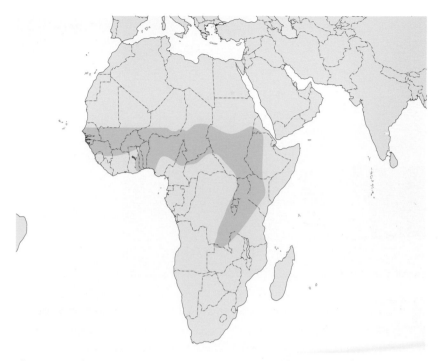

**Figure 11.1** The 'meningitis belt' of sub-Saharan Africa (shading) including countries with epidemic disease reported in the past 5 years.

Epidemic meningococcal disease in the meningitis belt of Africa is caused by serogroup A clones.

**Clinical syndromes.** Meningococcal infection may present clinically with features of meningitis (headache, nausea, nuchal rigidity, photophobia, fever, confusion, drowsiness), septicaemia (tachycardia, cold peripheries, prolonged capillary refill time, oliguria, tachypnoea, confusion, hypotension) or raised intracranial pressure (headache, seizures, focal signs, hypertension and bradycardia, pupillary changes, decreased level of consciousness). A characteristic non-blanching rash consisting of petechiae or purpura (Figure 11.2) occurs in more than 80% of cases.

**Therapy.** In most countries, meningococci remain susceptible to penicillins, cephalosporins and chloramphenicol, though there have been some reports of resistance developing. Data on local antibiotic sensitivities are important

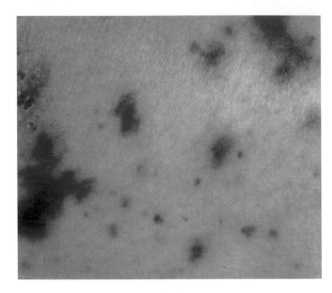

**Figure 11.2**
Meningococcal
rash.

in choosing appropriate therapy. When available, empirical treatment with
a high-dose, third-generation cephalosporin is recommended for suspected
meningococcal infection because the disease may be confused with
pneumococcal infection, in which penicillin resistance is more likely.
Third-generation cephalosporins are also recommended for cerebrospinal
fluid penetration.

The clinical imperative in managing individuals with meningococcal
infection is recognition and treatment of shock or raised intracranial
pressure.

**Prophylaxis** with antibiotics is recommended for household and kissing
contacts of those with meningococcal disease.

**Vaccines.** Meningococcal vaccine should be offered to travellers over 2 years
of age making an extended visit (> 1 month) to a hyperendemic or epidemic
area. In particular, those backpacking, living or working with local people,
or visiting remote parts of these areas should be offered the vaccine.
Vaccination is recommended for visitors to the meningitis belt. Individuals
with asplenia, complement deficiency and other immunosuppressing
conditions, including HIV infection, should also be vaccinated. Travellers to
Saudi Arabia for Umra, the Haj pilgrimage, and seasonal work must provide

evidence of vaccination against serogroups A and C meningococcus within 3 years. Although either of the available polysaccharide vaccines, A/C and A/C/Y/W135, was thought to be suitable, a large outbreak of serogroup W135 disease in 2000 was associated with the Haj and the quadrivalent vaccine is now preferable.

## Rabies

Rabies is an acute, invariably fatal encephalomyelitis. It is almost always transmitted via an infected-mammal bite, and an estimated 5–80% of such bites result in clinical disease if post-exposure prophylaxis is not administered. The greatest risk is when bites that bleed, are on the head and neck, or are from bats. Bites to the peripheries and those that do not break the skin have the lowest risk (see Table 11.3).

Epidemiology. Worldwide, rabies kills up to 60 000 people every year. The majority of reported deaths from rabies occur in Asia, particularly India and Bangladesh. Remaining deaths are reported mainly from the Philippines, Sri Lanka, Thailand, the Americas and Africa. Rabies is endemic worldwide, except in a few countries that the WHO has certified as rabies-free. However, many more countries can be considered rabies-free (Table 11.1).

Dogs are most often associated with transmission, and the majority of cases occur in countries with a large stray-dog population. In areas where rabies control measures are in place, such as North America and Europe, wild animals are the major rabies reservoirs (Table 11.2). In Europe, rabies occurs most frequently in Turkey and Romania; Turkey is the only European country in which dogs are a major reservoir for rabies. In Europe, the main reservoir is in the red fox, while in North America, most cases of rabies are associated with bats.

The at-risk population. Most dog bites occur in children under 10 years of age, because of their behaviour, size and inability to escape when attacked. Bites in children are more likely to involve the head and neck, whereas bites in adults are more likely on the peripheries.

Incubation period depends on the site and severity of the bite. It is usually less than 3 months, but can be as short as 7 days and as long as 6 years.

TABLE 11.1

**Areas not reporting rabies during 1996–1997 that can be considered rabies-free\***

| Region | Countries/territories |
| --- | --- |
| Africa | Cape Verde, Libya, Mauritius, Reunion, Seychelles |
| North America | Bermuda, St Pierre and Miquelon |
| Caribbean | Antigua and Barbuda, Aruba, Bahamas, Barbados, Cayman Islands, Guadeloupe, Jamaica, Martinique, Netherlands Antilles, St Kitts and Nevis, St Martin, St Vincent and Grenadines, Virgin Islands (UK and US) |
| South America | Uruguay |
| Asia | Bahrain, Brunei, Hong Kong, Indonesia (except Java, Kalimantan, Sumatra and Sulawesi), Japan, Kuwait, Malaysia-Sabah, Maldives, Qatar, Singapore, Taiwan |
| Europe | Albania, Cyprus, Denmark, Faroe Islands, Finland, Gibraltar, Greece, Iceland, Ireland, Isle of Man, Italy, Jersey, Macedonia, Malta, Monaco, Norway (mainland), Portugal, Spain (except Ceuta/Melilla), Sweden, UK |
| Oceania | American Samoa, Australia, Cook Islands, Fiji, French Polynesia, Guam, Kiribati, New Caledonia, New Zealand, Niue, Papua New Guinea, Solomon Islands, Tonga, Vanuatu |

\*Adapted from CDC, 1999–2000

**Clinical presentation.** The first symptoms are paraesthesiae, burning and pruritus at the site of the bite as the nervous system is invaded. Subsequently, the whole limb may become involved, and fever and anxiety typically develop. As the virus spreads, either encephalitic (furious, 70%) or paralytic (dumb, 30%) rabies may occur. Coma followed by death occurs within 2 days to 4 weeks of symptom onset.

**Diagnosis.** A fluorescent antibody test that detects rabies virus in corneal epithelial cells (from a corneal smear) or hair follicle cells (skin biopsy from the hairline) is available.

TABLE 11.2

**Rabies vectors**

- Badgers
- Bats
- Cats
- Cattle
- Cheetahs
- Coyotes
- Dogs
- Foxes

- Humans
- Jackals
- Lions
- Mongooses
- Monkeys
- Raccoons
- Skunks
- Wolves

**Prevention.** Potentially infected animals should be avoided, particularly by children. Parents and their children should be educated as part of their travel counselling. For individuals travelling to highly endemic areas, particularly where dogs are the main reservoir, pre-exposure prophylaxis should be considered (see Chapter 5).

### Post-exposure management

*Treatment of potentially infected wounds and bites* reduces transmission. Bites and wounds should be washed thoroughly and vigorously with soap and water, detergent or water alone, immediately. If available, a virucidal agent (such as 70% alcohol or iodine solution) should then be applied. The wound should not be sutured for 1–2 days if at all possible. Appropriate antibacterial and anti-tetanus measures should then be instituted.

*Vaccine prophylaxis* is almost completely effective in preventing rabies following exposure if undertaken early enough. However, it is reasonable to institute post-exposure prophylaxis even if 6 months have elapsed since exposure. Some authorities do not consider prophylaxis necessary if 12 months have expired. Vaccine may be administered to an exposed individual of any age and should not be withheld in pregnancy.

In previously unimmunized individuals with significant exposure, human diploid cell vaccine (HDCV) is administered on days 0, 3, 7, 14 and 28 (the standard Essen regimen) by intramuscular injection into the deltoid region (or thigh in a small child). The vaccine should never be injected into the gluteal region as the antibody response may be reduced. Human rabies immunoglobulin (HRIG) should be administered intramuscularly with the first dose of vaccine to provide protection until the host develops immunity. Half the HRIG dose should be infiltrated around the wound to neutralize virus in the tissues. A double first dose of vaccine is recommended for multiple severe bites in children.

In previously immunized individuals, where there has been clear documentation of complete pre-exposure immunization, HRIG is not required, but two booster doses of HDCV should be administered on days 0 and 3.

The WHO has classified the type of wound in developing recommendations for post-exposure prophylaxis (Table 11.3), but national guidelines vary and local sources should be sought.

TABLE 11.3

**Wound classification***

| Category | Level of exposure | Wound description | Treatment |
| --- | --- | --- | --- |
| I | None | Touching or feeding animals, or licks on intact skin | No treatment |
| II | Minor | Nibbling of uncovered skin Minor scratches or abrasions without bleeding Licks on broken skin | Local treatment plus HDCV (or alternative). Stop treatment if animal remains healthy after 10 days or is killed and proven to be rabies-free |
| III | Severe | Single or multiple transdermal bites or scratches Contamination of mucous membranes with saliva/licks | Local treatment HRIG/ERIG plus HDCV (or alternative) stop treatment if animal remains healthy after 10 days or is killed and proven to be rabies-free |

*Adapted from WHO, 1992

TABLE 11.4

**Vaccine schedules for post-exposure prophylaxis of rabies**

| Schedule | Vaccine | Route | Day of vaccination (number of doses at different sites) |
|---|---|---|---|
| Essen schedule | HDCV PVRV PCEC PDEV | Intramuscular | 0, 3, 7, 14, 28 |
| 2–1–1 schedule | HDCV PVRV PCEC PDEV | Intramuscular | 0 ($\times$ 2), 7, 21 |
| Two-site intradermal method | PVRV PCEC PDEV | Intradermal* | 0 ($\times$ 2), 3 ($\times$ 2), 7 ($\times$ 2), 28, 90 |
| Eight-site intradermal method | HDCV PCEC | Intradermal* | 0 ($\times$ 8), 4 ($\times$ 4), 28, 90 |

*The intradermal dose is one-fifth of the recommended intramuscular dose for each vaccine

*Alternative vaccines.* Several inactivated viral vaccines derived from cell culture are available for post-exposure prophylaxis, which are all equally effective and safe. In addition to HDCV, purified vero cell rabies vaccine (PVRV) has been used widely and has proven efficacy. Chicken embryo culture vaccine (PCEC) and duck embryo vaccine (PDEV) are also available in some countries. Unfortunately, many countries do not have safe inactivated purified cell culture or duck embryo vaccines available, but use brain tissue vaccines, which are cheaper to produce. The WHO recommends using suckling-mouse brain vaccine as an alternative when cell culture or embryo vaccines are unavailable.

Where HRIG is not available, purified equine rabies immunoglobulin (ERIG) is an alternative. However, there is a higher risk of anaphylaxis and serum sickness with this product.

*Alternative vaccine schedules.* The standard Essen regimen is the most widely used where sufficient supplies of vaccine are available (Table 11.4). However, a 2–1–1 regimen may also be used (two doses intramuscularly on day 0 in each arm, one dose on day 7 and one on day 21). If vaccines are in short supply, various immunogenic intradermal schedules can be used. Because the intradermal route is more difficult to deliver, intramuscular schedules are generally preferred.

**Deferring treatment.** When a bite is very unlikely to have transmitted rabies, it is reasonable to defer treatment for 48 hours if a definite negative diagnosis can be assured (by fluorescent antibody testing of the animal's brain). In the case of a vaccinated domestic animal, treatment may be deferred during 10 days of observation. If the animal shows any sign of illness in this time, vaccination should begin immediately. If fluorescent antibody testing of the brain of the animal that caused the bite is found to be rabies negative, post-exposure prophylaxis may then be discontinued.

## Sexually transmitted infections

Sexually transmitted infections (STIs) are a major public health problem in many areas frequented by travellers. In many countries, reliable STI prevalence data are lacking, and the high prevalences of certain STIs are often underestimated. Hepatitis B surface antigen (HBsAg) carriage rates, for example, are as high as 15% in some Asian, African and Pacific Island populations (compared with < 0.4% in the USA), and there are thought to be up to 300 million chronic carriers worldwide. In Papua New Guinea, up to 60 in every 1000 adults have an STI.

HIV infection is prevalent in many travel destinations, particularly sub-Saharan Africa; prevalence rates as high as 15–30% have been documented in some areas. In 1997, 13–25% of Thai prostitutes were HIV positive.

In addition to the increased risk of STIs, travellers may encounter infections different from those that exist in their home country. Lymphogranuloma venereum, chancroid, donovanosis, HIV-2 infection and HTLV-1 infection are prevalent in certain geographic regions, but uncommon in most western countries. Antibiotic resistance is also a major problem in some areas of the world. More than 50% of *Neisseria gonorrhoeae* isolates in some parts of Asia and Africa are resistant to penicillin.

Sexual contact with previously unknown partners is surprisingly common among travellers. STIs may be acquired from fellow travellers, sex workers and local inhabitants. Although much attention has been focused on the activities of 'sex tourists' (tourists who visit areas where sex is for sale), the majority of STIs in travellers occur outside this setting. Having said this, contact with prostitutes is associated with a high risk of acquiring STIs.

**Prevention.** Ideally, travellers should be counselled about the risk and prevention of STIs. Hepatitis B vaccination should be offered to travellers at risk, and the use of condoms emphasized. Travellers should also be made aware that condoms reduce, but do not eliminate, the risk of acquiring STIs. Furthermore, locally manufactured condoms may be of inferior quality.

Blood transfusions and needle sharing by intravenous drug users add to the risk of acquiring HIV infection. The safety of blood products cannot be guaranteed in many parts of the world. If transfusion is necessary in these areas, the blood should first be tested, if possible, for HIV antibodies.

## Viral hepatitis

Although many viruses can cause hepatitis, hepatitis A, B, C and E are most relevant to travellers.

**Hepatitis A** is transmitted via the faecal–oral route, and causes a typical acute hepatic illness after an incubation period of 15–50 days (typically about 4 weeks). The clinical severity can vary considerably from mild to severely debilitating. In young children (particularly those under 4 years of age), hepatitis A infection is usually asymptomatic. Chronic liver disease is a rare complication and the case-fatality rate is low. Hepatitis A infection may precipitate fulminant hepatitis in persons with concomitant hepatitis C infection.

Hepatitis A is endemic throughout most of the developing world (Figure 11.3) and is the vaccine-preventable infection most likely to be encountered by travellers. Infection is related to food and drink consumption in poorly sanitized settings, so travellers should avoid these. Safe and effective vaccines are now available and should be recommended to non-immune travellers to endemic areas. Alternatively immune globulin can be given, particularly if there is insufficient time to develop an antibody response. Travellers who think they have had hepatitis A infection in the

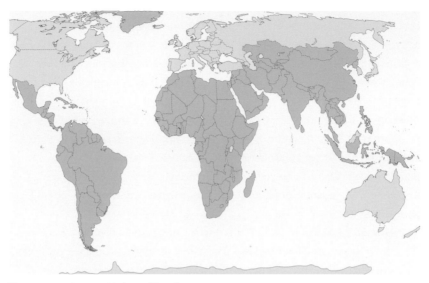

**Figure 11.3** Areas with hepatitis A in 1999–2000.

past can be tested for hepatitis A IgG antibodies; if present, they have lifelong immunity against reinfection.

**Hepatitis B** is transmitted by exchange of blood products or sexual activity. The incubation period is 6 weeks to 6 months, and clinical manifestations range from inapparent illness to fulminant hepatic necrosis and cirrhosis. The prevalence of chronic hepatitis B infection is high (≥ 8%) throughout much of the world (Figure 11.4). For most travellers, the risk of hepatitis B infection is low, and vaccination is recommended only for healthcare workers and for travellers likely to engage in risk activities.

**Hepatitis C** is transmitted mainly by exchange of blood products, though it can be transmitted through sexual activity. Acute infection is usually asymptomatic, but chronic carriage rates are high. The incubation period is 2 weeks to 6 months. The prevalence of hepatitis C is high in many parts of the world, and travellers at greatest risk are those exposed to blood products and engaging in high-risk sexual activities. No vaccine exists.

**Hepatitis E** is transmitted in a similar fashion and causes an illness similar to hepatitis A. Infection has been associated with particularly severe disease in pregnant women. Hepatitis E has been found in most parts of the developing world. Prevention is identical to that for hepatitis A, except that no vaccine is available and the efficacy of immune globulin is uncertain.

## Leptospirosis

Leptospirosis, caused by several serotypes of the spirochaete *Leptospira interrogans*, is endemic in the tropics and other parts of the world. Infection is transmitted indirectly through exposure to water or soil contaminated with urine from infected animals. Many animals can serve as reservoirs, with the major carriers varying between regions. Clinical manifestations include an acute generalized febrile illness, jaundice, renal failure, meningitis and pneumonitis.

Leptospirosis is of greatest risk to travellers undertaking water-based activities. Contact with potentially contaminated water should be minimized.

## Tuberculosis

Approximately one-third of the world's population is infected with tuberculosis, and two-thirds of these live in Asia. However, transmission

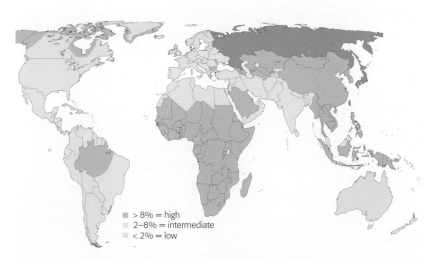

**Figure 11.4** Variations in the prevalence of hepatitis B. Adapted from CDC 1999–2000.

usually requires prolonged exposure to a coughing person with untreated pulmonary tuberculosis in a closed environment. Although there is little record of tuberculosis acquired by travellers, it is clear that, for most travellers, the risk is very low. Tuberculosis has been transmitted between passengers on commercial aircraft, but the risk appears to be no greater than for other confined spaces. The risk of transmission was greatest for those seated close to the index case. In those cases, exposure was prolonged (> 8 hours). No specific preventative measures are recommended. Travellers likely to be exposed to people with tuberculosis (e.g. healthcare workers) should know their tuberculin status prior to travel. The BCG vaccination is controversial, but it is probably effective against miliary tuberculosis and tuberculous meningitis in children and should therefore be considered for long-term travellers to Asia, Africa, and Central and South America.

## Tetanus

Tetanus is a worldwide problem and may occur in an unvaccinated person anywhere in the world. The pre-travel clinic provides an ideal opportunity to ensure tetanus vaccination is current.

## Diphtheria

Diphtheria remains a problem in much of the world. Large outbreaks occurred throughout the former USSR following breakdown of the immunization programme. Diphtheria vaccine is usually administered in combination with tetanus vaccine.

## Influenza

Influenza epidemics occur annually in temperate regions during the winter and spring months. The season is usually from November to March in the northern hemisphere, and from May to October in the southern hemisphere. Influenza can occur year round in the tropics. The travellers' risk depends on the travel destination and the time of year. Vaccination should be considered for travellers over 65 years of age, and those with chronic lung or cardiac conditions travelling to areas with ongoing influenza transmission. Recently, influenza outbreaks amongst travellers have been associated particularly with cruise ships.

CHAPTER 12
# Environmental and climatic factors

## Motor-vehicle accidents

The most frequent cause of travel-associated death is trauma, usually due to motor-vehicle accidents. In many countries, roads are crowded and in poor condition, motor vehicles are poorly maintained, and seat belts are often missing. Consumption of drugs and alcohol, unfamiliarity with traffic regulations or vehicles in different countries, long journey times and inadequate sleep are significant factors in many serious and fatal accidents. In addition, travellers often take risks that they would not consider in their home countries, such as not wearing helmets while riding motorcycles and riding in the back of open vehicles. Motorcycles carry the greatest risk.

To minimize the risk of motor vehicle accidents, travellers should be advised to:
• avoid riding motorcycles
• check the condition of motor vehicles they intend to travel in
• wear seat belts
• avoid alcohol consumption if driving
• avoid excessive speed
• avoid driving at night.

## Heat- and sun-related illnesses

Travellers to tropical and sub-tropical countries are susceptible to a number of specific heat- or sun-related medical problems. These conditions may also affect travellers to colder climates where sun exposure is high, for example during a skiing holiday.

Sunburn. Ultraviolet (UV) light damages the skin, causing burning, 'ageing' and neoplasia. Travellers should avoid exposure at the hottest times of day, and use clothing, sunblock creams and lotions. For individuals who wish to expose their skin to UV radiation, sunblock creams that filter UVA and UVB with a sun protection factor (SPF) of at least 25 should be used.

Particular care regarding protection from the sun should be taken whilst on or in the sea and lakes, or on snow as reflected rays lead to increased exposure to UV radiation.

**Snowblindness** is sunburn of the cornea and conjunctiva caused by intense solar radiation being reflected from snow. It is intensely painful, and best treated with a combination of non-steroidal anti-inflammatory drugs, chloramphenicol eye lotion and a cycloplegic agent such as 1% cyclopentolate. Wearing sunglasses with a UV filter can prevent snowblindness.

**Minor heat-related illnesses** are troublesome for travellers, but can usually be resolved with oral rehydration alone. Heat exhaustion and heatstroke, on the other hand, are more serious and require prompt recognition and treatment. Most of these conditions are avoided by maintaining adequate hydration (Table 12.1).

**Heat exhaustion** is caused by loss of salt and water through sweating, and inadequate replacement of one or both of these. It typically affects those who travel to hot climates and then exercise more than usual. It is characterized by sweating, syncope, headache, dizziness, malaise, myalgia fatigue and hypovolaemia. Heat exhaustion is managed by oral rehydration and simple skin cooling, but occasionally patients require hospitalization and intravenous therapy. Maintaining adequate hydration before and during exposure to heat stress prevents heat exhaustion.

**Heatstroke** is a serious medical emergency resulting from loss of normal temperature control mechanisms. The condition mainly affects healthy young men who engage in strenuous exercise in a hot climate, and the elderly. It is characterized by initial symptoms of heat exhaustion followed by loss of sweating, changes in mental state, headache, gastrointestinal disturbance and extreme elevation of body temperature. Neurological abnormalities distinguish heatstroke from heat exhaustion. Untreated, there may be a rapid progression to multi-organ failure, coma and death. Management of heatstroke is by rapid reduction of core temperature to prevent organ and particularly central nervous system damage. First-aid

TABLE 12.1

**Heat-related illnesses**

| Condition | Symptoms | Treatment |
|---|---|---|
| Heat cramps | Cramps in limb muscles | Oral fluid and salt replacement |
| Heat oedema | Skin oedema | Self-limiting |
| Heat syncope | Syncope due to vasodilatation and blood pooling | Fluid replacement and cooling |
| Heat tetany | Carpopedal spasm and perioral paraesthesiae | Oral fluid and salt replacement |
| Prickly heat | Pruritic vesicles | Chlorhexidine lotion/cream |
| Heat exhaustion | Sweating, syncope, myalgia, fatigue, hyperventilation, tachycardia, hypotension | Oral rehydration and cooling |
| Heat stroke | Hyperthermia, headache, central nervous system and gastrointestinal disturbance, tachycardia, ataxia, delirium, coma, hyperventilation, hepatitis, acute renal failure, rhabdomyolysis | Urgent skin surface cooling Intensive care management |

management is surface cooling followed by invasive methods of cooling in hospital and management of the widespread secondary effects of the hyperthermia. Dehydration is not necessarily a major component of heatstroke. If an individual exposed to a hot climate allows sufficient time to acclimatize before undertaking strenuous activity, limits the amount of activity in a non-air-conditioned environment and takes regular breaks to cool off between episodes of activity, heatstroke can probably be prevented.

**Other heat-related illnesses.** In addition to specific heat-related illness, morbidity and mortality due to non-heat-related illnesses, particularly cardiovascular, cerebrovascular, renal and respiratory diseases, increases during 'heatwaves'. In most conditions, dehydration is assumed to play a role in the patient's deterioration. Thus patients with these underlying medical problems should be advised of the importance of maintaining adequate hydration in hot climates.

## Cold-related illness

Cold environments exist in many popular travel destinations, particularly skiing destinations. However, cold injury in this group of travellers is unusual. Significant cold injury occurs mainly amongst hikers, backpackers and climbers who are caught in deteriorating weather conditions and are inadequately prepared.

**Hypothermia** is defined as a fall in core body temperature below 35°C. Overall, the elderly and young children are at greatest risk, but these are groups unlikely to be exposed to the cold. Most cases of hypothermia occur as a result of cold exposure during hiking, mountaineering or water sports.

Use of adequate and appropriate clothing in potentially cold environments can prevent hypothermia. Climbers and hikers travelling to remote mountain or wilderness areas should seek expert clothing advice. Warm, waterproof and windproof garments are essential. Hikers should also consider their requirements should they get lost, caught in bad weather or benighted in the wilderness. For those on water-sports holidays, advice about water temperatures and appropriate wet/dry suits and other clothing is essential, as body temperature can fall rapidly following immersion in cold water.

*Mild hypothermia* results in shivering and changes in central nervous system function, such as loss of judgement and mild ataxia, and is characterized by a core temperature of 32–35°C. Severe confusion may occur below 33°C. Treatment consists of prevention of further heat loss (insulation from the ground, protection from the wind and removal of wet clothes), active external rewarming (shared body heat or warming packs applied centrally) and correction of hypogylcaemia with warm, sweet drinks.

*Severe hypothermia.* The clinical features of severe hypothermia depend on core temperature. As core temperature falls below 32°C, shivering ceases, and there is profound hypoventilation and bradycardia, loss of reflexes and fixed dilated pupils, and the victim may appear dead. Severe hypothermia is best managed in an intensive care unit. Moving a casualty with severe hypothermia can be problematic as inappropriate attempts at cardiopulmonary resuscitation, changes in posture and jarring during evacuation may convert life-sustaining bradycardia to ventricular fibrillation. If there is no hope of transfer to a hospital, after prevention of further heat loss, external warming is the only practical solution.

**Frostbite** results from freezing of tissues. It most commonly affects the digits, distal limbs, nose and ears, so in a cold environment, any factor that decreases the blood supply to these areas will increase the risk of frostbite. Travellers should be advised to acquire well-fitting boots and to wear appropriately insulated gloves and footwear in cold environments. Individuals with Raynaud's phenomenon are at particular risk.

Frostbite is treated by rapid rewarming with water at 40°C when circumstances are such that refreezing will not occur. It should ideally be undertaken in hospital. It is essential to avoid refreezing or causing further tissue damage by rubbing or other trauma to the damaged skin. Surgery should be delayed until the fingers are mummified and there is a clear line of surgical demarcation. This may take several months.

## Altitude illness

Altitude sickness is a risk for travellers above 2500 m. The number of people travelling to such altitudes has increased dramatically in recent decades, many of whom lack adequate knowledge and preparation about the potential dangers of high-altitude exposure (Table 12.2).

Acclimatization is the process by which the body gradually adjusts to high-altitude hypoxia. Several physiological changes occur that increase oxygen delivery to the tissues, including increased ventilation and haemoglobin concentration. Acclimatization to high altitude is possible up to about 5500 m.

**Acute mountain sickness (AMS)** is the result of rapid ascent to altitudes over 2500 m without allowing sufficient time for acclimatization. It is probably a mild form of hypoxia-induced cerebral oedema. AMS is a constellation of symptoms, including headache, nausea, vomiting, fatigue, anorexia, dizziness and sleep disturbance. These symptoms can be severe and are usually unpleasant, and can seriously restrict the enjoyment of the holiday. The incidence of AMS depends on the rate of ascent and the final altitude

TABLE 12.2

**Types of altitude sickness and their treatments**

| Altitude sickness | Symptoms | Prevention | Treatment |
|---|---|---|---|
| Acute mountain sickness (AMS) | Headache, nausea, vomiting, fatigue, anorexia, dizziness, sleep disturbance | Slow ascent rate of 300 m/day above 3000 m OR acetazolamide 250 mg twice daily | Mild: analgesia (paracetamol/ acetaminophen) Severe: descent Dexamethasone 4 mg four times daily Oxygen Hyperbaric chamber |
| High-altitude cerebral oedema (HACE) | Ataxia, behavioural changes, hallucinations, disorientation, confusion, coma, death | As for AMS | Descent Oxygen Dexamethasone 4 mg four times daily Hyperbaric chamber |
| High-altitude pulmonary oedema (HAPE) | Dyspnoea, reduced exercise tolerance, dry cough, blood-stained sputum, crackles on auscultation cases | Graded ascent as for AMS Nifedipine 20 mg slow release 8 hourly in recurrent cases | Descent Oxygen Nifedipine SR 20 mg four times daily Hyperbaric chamber |

gained. Approximately half of all trekkers ascending to 5400 m in Nepal develop AMS.

*Prevention* involves a slow, graded ascent. Over 3000 m, AMS is unlikely to occur with an ascent rate of 300 m per day. Trekking schedules that allow a slow ascent and a rest day every 3 days or 1000 m should be sought where possible. Prophylaxis with acetazolamide, taken from the day before ascent above 2500 m, is effective in preventing AMS. However, side-effects include allergic reactions, paraesthesiae and mild diuresis, so acetazolamide should probably be reserved for individuals who need to make a rapid ascent. A test run at sea level prior to travel is a good idea as some individuals find the drug intolerable.

*Treatment.* Most individuals who develop AMS have mild illness that is treatable with simple analgesia (paracetamol/acetaminophen). AMS sufferers should not continue to ascend, but instead remain with companions until symptoms have resolved and acclimatization occurred. Ascent can then recommence. Descent is the only definitive therapy.

Portable hyperbaric chambers, consisting of an airtight bag inflated to above atmospheric pressure to simulate a lower altitude, are now carried by many organized trekking groups. If descent is not undertaken after treatment with this equipment, AMS symptoms are likely to recur.

**High-altitude cerebral oedema (HACE)** occurs in a small proportion of trekkers to high altitude (< 1%). The condition is usually preceded by AMS symptoms, and features include ataxia, behavioural changes, hallucinations, disorientation, confusion, and eventually coma and death. Ataxia is a prominent feature in many cases, and is often the last to resolve.

HACE is prevented by careful acclimatization. If symptoms or signs of HACE develop, descent is imperative as there is a high mortality. Therapy with oxygen, use of a portable hyperbaric chamber or dexamethasone may all facilitate descent, but should never be allowed to delay descent.

**High-altitude pulmonary oedema (HAPE).** About 1% of high-altitude travellers develop HAPE. This form of pulmonary oedema seems to consist of hypoxia-induced pulmonary hypertension and capillary leakiness. Clinical features of this disorder include dyspnoea, reduced exercise tolerance, dry cough, blood-stained sputum and crackles on auscultation. HAPE is prevented by slow ascent and may be more likely in individuals suffering from an intercurrent viral illness. HAPE can be rapidly fatal.

HAPE is treated effectively by descent. Oxygen and simulated descent in a portable hyperbaric chamber may facilitate, but should never delay descent. Nifedipine has been found to be a useful treatment for HAPE and should be used to facilitate descent in individuals with this condition. It is also a useful prophylactic for those with a history of recurrent HAPE.

## Diving-related illness

Travellers to many destinations undertake casual diving without receiving adequate instruction. However, serious consequences of diving and decompression may occur even during/after shallow dives. For the novice or inexperienced diver, a qualified instructor should be available for training and supervision. A medical examination by a diving-medicine physician is advisable as there are a number of contraindications to diving (Table 12.3).

**Barotrauma** to any air-filled spaces can occur as changes in ambient pressure during ascent and descent alter the volume of the trapped gas. The most commonly affected areas are the sinuses, middle/inner ear and the lung. Dental and gastric barotrauma have also been described.

*Middle-ear barotrauma* is caused by inward compression of the tympanic membrane during descent or expansion of air in the middle ear during ascent. It can be prevented by adequate training in middle-ear pressure

TABLE 12.3

**Relative and absolute contraindications to diving**

- Acute upper or lower respiratory infection or allergy
- Poorly controlled diabetes mellitus
- Drug addiction or intoxication
- Emphysema
- Epilepsy
- Impaired respiratory function
- Obesity
- Perforated tympanic membrane
- Pregnancy
- Pulmonary cysts
- Psychiatric illness
- Recent myocardial infarction
- Spontaneous pneumothoraces
- Syncope

equalization techniques and by not diving during upper respiratory tract infections. In some individuals with recurrent problems, topical or system vasoconstrictors can be used. When middle-ear barotrauma occurs, the prominent symptom is pain, but deafness and vertigo may also occur and rarely facial nerve palsy. The condition is usually self-resolving.

*Inner-ear barotrauma* is due to pressure on or rupture of the oval and round windows, usually during descent. Rupture of these membranes results in sudden onset of nausea and vomiting, tinnitus, vertigo and deafness. Specialist advice is required.

*Sinus barotrauma* occurs during descent and is associated particularly with upper respiratory tract infections. It most commonly affects the frontal sinuses and results in sinus pain and bleeding. Maxillary sinus barotrauma can result in trigeminal nerve palsy (facial paraesthesiae). Sinus barotrauma usually resolves spontaneously with equalization.

*Dental barotrauma.* Expansion of trapped gas in the pulp of a tooth can cause dental pain and dislodge a filling.

*Gastric barotrauma.* Expansion of swallowed air in the stomach can cause pain and even gastric rupture during ascent. Carbonated drinks and large meals should be avoided before diving.

*Pulmonary barotrauma* (pulmonary overpressurization syndrome, POPS) is due to air expansion in the lungs during a rapid ascent, and is associated particularly with breath-holding during ascent or underlying pulmonary disease. Expansion of gas in the lungs can result in pneumothorax, pneumomediastinum, subcutaneous emphysema and/or arterial gas embolism (if air ruptures into a blood vessel). In most cases, management of pneumothorax, subcutaneous emphysema and pneumomediastinum is conservative. Large collections of intrapleural air need decompression with a chest drain.

**Arterial gas embolism** occurs when bubbles of gas, expanded during ascent, rupture into blood vessels. It may occur even after very brief shallow dives. The gas embolizes to distant arterioles and capillaries, causing occlusion. Common sites are the brain, coronary arteries and spinal cord, and the diver may suffer neurological symptoms (such as coma, seizures, paralysis and focal neurology) or symptoms of myocardial infarction. Gas embolism should be suspected in a diver who has made a rapid ascent and then

TABLE 12.4

**Types of decompression sickness**

| Type | Symptoms | Treatment |
|------|----------|-----------|
| I | Skin rash, pruritus and/or muscle/ joint pain | Recompression or observe |
| II | Neurological, vestibular or cardiopulmonary | 100% oxygen and recompression |

becomes unconscious. Immediate recompression is necessary as well as other supportive measures.

**Decompression sickness** is associated with longer deep dives and rapid ascent (Table 12.4). Nitrogen dissolves into the tissues during the dive and bubbles of nitrogen form on reascent. The bubbles are typically venous but also form in the skin, joints, muscles and nerves giving symptoms of 'the bends'.

Mild decompression sickness should be treated with recompression where possible, but as the condition can resolve spontaneously, a period of observation is reasonable when this is not possible. In severe decompression sickness, oxygen therapy and recompression should be initiated urgently. Decompression sickness may develop during rapid ascent from sea level to altitude or after a dive. In most cases, air travel should be delayed for 12–24 hours.

**Diving gas toxicity.** Hyperbaric oxygen in diving mixtures may produce cerebral toxicity with resulting nausea, hallucinations and paraesthesiae. Convulsions may also occur, which can have serious consequences while diving. Returning to normal air breathing at the surface should allow resolution of symptoms, as long as pulmonary barotrauma has not occurred during ascent. Nitrogen (and other inert gases) induces narcosis during diving that disappears during decompression. Replacing nitrogen with helium in gas mixtures can reduce the risk. Diving gas mixtures may be contaminated with carbon monoxide prior to use, resulting in headache and malaise, a flushed appearance, followed by coma and death. Treatment is with 100% oxygen. Carbon dioxide may build up with certain diving breathing systems resulting in dyspnoea, headaches, seizures, coma and death. At this stage, ascent will increase the percentage of carbon dioxide and cause a deterioration in clinical status. Initial management consists of trying to reduce carbon dioxide production by reducing activity, and increasing carbon dioxide removal by controlled breathing. It may be necessary to change to an open-circuit breathing system.

**Immersion pulmonary oedema.** Some individuals develop pulmonary oedema following immersion in water as a result of central redistribution of blood. Thought to be associated with an exaggerated vasoconstrictor response to cold, poor left ventricular function and later development of hypertension, immersion pulmonary oedema can occur at all ages and usually develops soon after immersion. After removal from the water, it resolves spontaneously.

## Venomous bites and stings

Life threatening bites and stings are extremely rare. Knowledge about local venomous creatures and their habitats allows strategies for avoidance.

**Hymenoptera.** Bees, wasps and hornets rarely cause serious direct toxicity as a result of their venom. Anaphylaxis from such stings is a risk in those with hypersensitivity. When this condition is recognized, adrenaline (epinephrine) should be carried.

**Snakes.** Most snakebites do not involve venom that is dangerous to humans, but some species can inject sufficient venom to be lethal. Most of the bites occur on the limbs. Treatment consists of reassurance, immobilization of the affected limb, analgesia and immediate hospital medical advice. All other treatments and remedies should be avoided. Anti-venom is indicated if there are signs of spontaneous bleeding (mucous membranes, haematuria), neurological signs, cardiovascular compromise or swelling of more than half the bitten limb. Unless the species can be identified, a polyvalent anti-venom that covers the locally prevalent species should be used. Anaphylaxis is a major risk after administration of anti-venom, and adrenaline (epinephrine) should be available. If toxic effects of snakebites do occur, supportive therapy may be necessary to manage haemorrhage, respiratory paralysis, cardiovascular collapse and secondary infection.

**Marine animals.** Many species of fish and jellyfish, as well as some octopuses, are poisonous. Local knowledge is important in avoiding contact with these creatures. Venomous tentacles or spines should be removed as soon as possible and complications, including arrhythmias and respiratory paralysis, managed appropriately. Immersing the affected limb in warm water at 45°C inactivates the venom from stingray spines, while vinegar inactivates the nematocysts of box jellyfish and prevents discharge of venom.

**Scorpions and spiders.** Scorpion stings are not usually fatal except in children, but are very painful and can lead to catecholamine release. Dangerous scorpions are found in India, Africa, the Middle East, and North, South and Central America.

Spider bites are unpleasant but are rarely life-threatening, except in children. Anti-venom is available in some countries for dangerous species. The most dangerous are the black widow spider, banana and funnel web spiders, which can both cause cardiovascular compromise and neurological symptoms, and the brown recluse spider, which causes local necrosis, coagulopathy and haemoglobinuria. Poisonous spiders are also found in Australia, South Africa, Mediterranean countries and North, South and Central America.

CHAPTER 13
# Returned travellers

Travellers may seek medical attention on returning to their home country. Although most problems travellers may present with are minor or self-limiting, a small proportion return with potentially life-threatening infections. In addition, screening for some infections is recommended in certain asymptomatic returned travellers.

Several issues peculiar to travel need to be addressed when assessing illness in returned travellers.

- The areas the traveller has visited, including stopovers, are critical and will help determine which infections are part of the differential diagnosis, and which can be excluded.
- The time interval between potential exposure and development of symptoms can be useful for excluding some infections. For example, an incubation period of more than 3 weeks will exclude many arboviral infections.
- The time of year of travel is important as some infections, such as Japanese encephalitis, are transmitted seasonally.
- The individual's vaccination and drug history are important considerations.
- Risk behaviour undertaken while travelling, such as sexual activity, blood transfusions and swimming in fresh water in Africa, can provide clues to certain infections.

The most common presenting symptoms in returned travellers are diarrhoea and fever, in that order. Skin complaints, sexually transmitted infections and respiratory symptoms are also common.

## Diarrhoea

Infectious diarrhoea is very common among travellers returning from certain countries. It is useful to distinguish acute diarrhoea from chronic diarrhoea (lasting 4 or more weeks) as the likely pathogens differ. Most travellers' diarrhoea is acute, lasting less than 1 week (see Chapter 8). Parasitic infections are the most common cause of chronic diarrhoea in returned travellers, and some bacteria can also cause persisting diarrhoea (Table 13.1). However, not all chronic diarrhoea has an infectious aetiology.

Initial evaluation should include faecal studies for bacteria and parasites. Although most enteric pathogens are detected in the first faeces specimen examined, at least three specimens should be sent to achieve acceptable sensitivity. If no faecal pathogens are detected and the diarrhoea has

TABLE 13.1

**Aetiology of diarrhoea in the returning traveller**

**Bacteria**

- *Campylobacter* spp.
- *Aeromonas hydrophila*
- *Pleisiomonas shigelloides*
- *Clostridium difficile*
- Multiple episodes of acute bacterial diarrhoea (i.e. not truly chronic)

**Protozoa**

- *Giardia lamblia*
- *Entamoeba histolytica*
- *Cryptosporidium parvum*
- *Cyclospora cayatenensis*

**Helminths**

- *Schistosoma mansoni*
- *Schistosoma japonicum*
- Hookworm
- *Strongyloides stercoralis*
- *Capillaria philippinensis*

**Tropical sprue**

**Non-infectious causes**

- Disaccharidase deficiency
- Drugs (including antimicrobials)
- Irritable bowel syndrome

TABLE 13.2

**Aetiology of fever in returning travellers**

| Incubation period | | | |
|---|---|---|---|
| **< 10 days** | **10–21 days** | **> 21 days** | **Variable** |
| • Dengue | • Malaria | • Malaria | • Drug fever |
| • Enteric fever (particularly paratyphoid fever) | • Enteric fever | • Hepatitis A–E | |
| | • Typhus | • Brucellosis | |
| • Typhus (particularly tick typhus) | • Hepatitis A and E | • Visceral leishmaniasis | |
| | • Leptospirosis | | |
| | • African trypanosomiasis | • Rabies | |
| • Yellow fever | • Chagas' disease | • Acute schistosomiasis | |
| • Legionellosis | • Q fever | • Tuberculosis | |
| • Relapsing fever | • Relapsing fever | • Extraintestinal amoebiasis | |
| • Plague | • Arthropod-borne encephalitides | • Melioidosis | |
| • Arthropod borne encephalitides | | • Filariasis | |
| | • Brucellosis | • Acute HIV infection | |
| • Bacterial sepsis | • Melioidosis | | |
| • Influenza | | | |

persisted for more than 3–4 weeks, lower gastrointestinal endoscopy and mucosal biopsy may be indicated.

## Fever

Fever in the returning traveller may be attributable to a wide variety of infections. In many cases, fever is part of a non-specific illness and is unaccompanied by focal symptoms. As part of the initial evaluation, an accurate exposure history is essential. Some important causes of fever in returned travellers can be differentiated according to their incubation periods (Table 13.2). Malaria, enteric fever, hepatitis A and dengue are relatively common in travellers returning from the tropics. Malaria and enteric fever require particular attention as each can present with a non-specific febrile illness, and result in serious, life-threatening complications.

**Malaria** should be considered in any traveller returning with fever. If exposure to malaria is possible, a blood film should be made and examined within the same day, particularly if the patient is unwell. If the initial blood film is negative and suspicion of malaria remains high, films should be repeated every 6–12 hours for up to 2 days. As the signs and symptoms of malaria are non-specific and delaying treatment of falciparum malaria can have disastrous consequences, the threshold for testing for malaria should be low.

**Typhoid fever** frequently presents with non-specific symptoms and signs. Fever may be accompanied by constipation, diarrhoea, respiratory or neuropsychiatric symptoms. Current typhoid vaccinations are no more than 70% effective and, consequently, previous typhoid vaccination does not exclude this diagnosis. Blood and stool cultures are an important part of the diagnostic work-up of all types of suspected enteric fevers, including typhoid and paratyphoid fevers.

### Eosinophilia

The most common causes of peripheral eosinophilia in the returned traveller are invasive helminthic infections and allergic conditions (Table 13.3). Eosinophilia is occasionally associated with infection with the coccidian parasite, *Isospora belli*; otherwise, eosinophilia is not associated with protozoan infections, including malaria, toxoplasmosis, giardiasis and amoebiasis.

The initial diagnostic evaluation includes stool, urine and, if filariasis is a possibility, blood microscopy for parasites. If these tests are negative, and exposure histories are suggestive, serological testing for schistosomiasis, filariasis and toxocariasis may be appropriate. Interpretation of serological tests can be complicated by cross-reactions and the inability to distinguish active from past infection. However, in travellers normally resident in areas where these parasites are not endemic, serological testing can be useful. Examination of biopsy material may also be indicated for certain infections, such as rectal mucosa (schistosomiasis), skin (onchocerciasis) and muscle (trichinosis). Examination of cerebrospinal fluid is essential in cases of suspected eosinophilic meningitis.

TABLE 13.3

**Causes of eosinophilia**

| Parasitic causes | Non-parasitic causes |
|---|---|
| • Nematodes | • Allergies |
| – ascariasis | – atopic dermatitis |
| – hookworm infection | – urticaria |
| – strongyloidiasis | • Drugs |
| – lymphatic filariasis | – penicillins |
| – onchocerciasis | – tetracyclines |
| – loiasis | – non-steroidal anti-inflammatory drugs |
| – angiostrongyliasis | – allopurinol |
| – visceral larva migrans (toxocariasis) | – phenytoin |
| – trichinellosis | – aspirin |
| – dracunculiasis | • Neoplasms |
| • Trematodes | lymphomas |
| – schistosomiasis | – some leukaemias |
| – fascioliasis | – other malignancies |
| – fasciopsiasis | • Infections |
| – paragonimiasis | – tuberculosis |
| – clonorchiasis | – coccidioidomycosis |
| | – bronchopulmonary aspergillosis |
| | • Others |
| | – hypereosinophilic syndromes |
| | – pemphigus |

## Jaundice

Viral hepatitis, particularly caused by hepatitis A virus, is the most common cause of jaundice in travellers. Hepatitis E virus is prevalent in many parts of the world and is transmitted in a similar fashion to hepatitis A. Unprotected sexual contact and blood transfusion are risk factors for acquiring hepatitis

127

B infection. Infections with Epstein-Barr virus, yellow fever virus, cytomegalovirus, dengue fever virus, *Leptospira*, *Coxiella burnettii*, and many other agents can cause acute hepatitis. Malaria, drug reactions (e.g. to sulfur-containing antimalarials) and biliary tract disease can underlie jaundice. Initial diagnostic work-up should include liver function tests and serology for the agents of viral hepatitis.

## The asymptomatic returned traveller

There are several indications for screening asymptomatic returned travellers. Such circumstances include travellers who:

- have had moderate- to high-risk exposure to certain infections
- have been living overseas for a long period of time, generally more than 6 months
- wish to be screened.

### Travellers encountering potential exposure to certain infections

*Sexually transmitted infections.* If appropriate, genital and other smears should be taken for microscopy and culture. Serological testing should be performed for syphilis, HIV and hepatitis B.

*Blood transfusions.* Travellers who received blood products of uncertain quality while travelling should be screened for transmissible viruses (HIV, hepatitis B and hepatitis C), and malaria if symptoms are suggestive.

*Schistosomiasis.* The urine and stools of travellers who have swum in freshwater bodies in Africa and parts of Asia should be screened for schistosomiasis. Results may be negative during the first 2–3 months following exposure in the presence of infection. If negative, the test should be repeated after a month.

*Gastrointestinal pathogens* usually cause symptomatic disease, most commonly diarrhoea. Some parasitic infections may cause little, if any, symptoms by the time the traveller has returned home. For asymptomatic returned travellers concerned that they may have acquired an infection, stool samples can be examined. In returned travellers who are well and who do not have diarrhoea, bacterial stool cultures are of little, if any, value.

### Evaluating the returned long-term traveller

When appropriate, the following tests should be considered:

- peripheral blood; full blood count, including eosinophil count, and liver function tests
- microscopic stool examination for parasites
- tuberculin skin test to document tuberculin conversion
- serological testing for STIs, transfusion transmissible viruses and parasites as appropriate
- chest X-ray for tuberculosis.

# Appendix A

## Internet resources

American Society for Tropical Medicine and Hygiene at
**www.astmh.org**

Centers for Disease Control and Prevention at
**www.cdc.gov**

International Society for Travel Medicine at
**www.istm.org**

International Society for Mountain Medicine at
**www.medicine.mc.duke.edu/ismm/**

International Association of Medical Assistance for Travellers at
**www.sentex.net/~iamat/**

Travel Health online at
**www.tripprep.com**

World Health Organization at
**who.int**

Canada's CDC at
**hwcweb.hwc.ca/hpb/lcdc/new_e.html**

Traveller's Advisory Service at
**www.masta.org/**

Association for Safe International Road Travel at
**www.asirt.org**

Divers Alert Network (DAN) at
**www.diversalertnetwork.org**

# Appendix B

## Vaccines, malaria risk, travellers' diarrhoea risk and endemic diseases by country

Vaccines are listed that are either recommended or suggested for each country. Some vaccines are recommended only for particular groups or activities. Details of vaccine indications are given in Table 5.1 and in other sections of this book.

Key:
C, clonorchiasis; Dr, dracunculiasis; D, dengue; Fa, fasciolopsiasis; F, filariasis; H, viral haemorrhagic fevers other than dengue; L, leishmaniasis; O, onchocerciasis; P, plague; Pa, paragonomiasis; S, schistosomiasis; Ti, tick typhus, sometimes recommended

| | Hepatitis A vaccine recommended | Japanese encephalitis vaccine recommended | Japanese encephalitis endemic areas | Poliomyelitis vaccine recommended | Typhoid vaccine recommended | Typhoid vaccine recommended for some travellers | Yellow fever — Vaccine required | Yellow fever — Vaccine recommended for some travellers | Yellow fever — Vaccine required if travelling from certain areas | Malaria — Malarious areas present | Malaria — Chloroquine resistance | Rabies-free or not recently reported | Tick-borne encephalitis present in some areas | Other endemic diseases |
|---|---|---|---|---|---|---|---|---|---|---|---|---|---|---|
| Afghanistan | ✓ | | | ✓ | ✓ | | | | ✓ | ✓ | ✓ | | | H,L,Ti |
| Albania | ✓ | | | ✓ | ✓ | | | | ✓ | ✓ | | ✓ | ✓ | L,Ti |
| Algeria | ✓ | | | ✓ | ✓ | | | | ✓ | ✓ | | | | S |
| American Samoa | ✓ | | | ✓ | ✓ | | | | ✓ | | | ✓ | | F,D |
| Andorra | | | | | | ✓ | | | | | | | | |
| Angola | ✓ | | | ✓ | | ✓ | | ✓ | ✓ | ✓ | ✓ | | | F,H,O,P,S |
| Antigua & Barbuda | ✓ | | | | | | | | ✓ | | | ✓ | | D |
| Argentina | ✓ | | | | | | | | | ✓ | | | | |

131

| Country | Hepatitis A vaccine recommended | Japanese encephalitis vaccine recommended | Japanese encephalitis endemic areas | Poliomyelitis vaccine recommended | Typhoid vaccine recommended | Typhoid vaccine recommended for some travellers | Yellow fever: Vaccine required | Yellow fever: Vaccine recommended for some travellers | Yellow fever: Vaccine required if travelling from certain areas | Malaria: Malarious areas present | Malaria: Chloroquine resistance | Rabies-free or not recently reported | Tick-borne encephalitis present in some areas | Other endemic diseases |
|---|---|---|---|---|---|---|---|---|---|---|---|---|---|---|
| Armenia | ✓ | | | | ✓ | | | | | ✓ | | | | |
| Australia | | | | | | | | | ✓ | | | ✓ | | |
| Austria | | | | | | | | | | | | | ✓ | |
| Azerbaijan | ✓ | | | | ✓ | | | | | ✓ | | | | |
| Bahamas | ✓ | | | | ✓ | | | | ✓ | | | ✓ | | D |
| Bahrain | ✓ | ✓ | | ✓ | ✓ | | | | | | | ✓ | | L |
| Bangladesh | ✓ | | | ✓ | ✓ | | | | ✓ | ✓ | ✓ | | | D,F,L |
| Barbados | ✓ | | | ✓ | ✓ | | | | ✓ | | | ✓ | | D |
| Belarus | ✓ | | | | ✓ | | | | | | | | | |
| Belgium | | | | | | | | | | | | | | |
| Belize | ✓ | | ✓ | ✓ | ✓ | | ✓ | | ✓ | ✓ | | | | D,L,T |
| Benin | ✓ | | ✓ | ✓ | ✓ | ✓ | | ✓ | | ✓ | ✓ | | | F,H,O,S,T,Ti |
| Bermuda | | | | | | | | | | | | ✓ | | D |
| Bhutan | ✓ | ✓ | | | ✓ | ✓ | | | ✓ | ✓ | ✓ | | | D,F,L |
| Bolivia | ✓ | | | ✓ | ✓ | | | | | ✓ | ✓ | | | L,P,T |
| Bosnia-Herzegovina | ✓ | | | | ✓ | | | | | | | | | |
| Botswana | ✓ | | | ✓ | ✓ | | | | ✓ | ✓ | ✓ | | | H,S,T,Ti |
| Brazil | ✓ | | | | ✓ | ✓ | | ✓ | ✓ | ✓ | ✓ | | | D,L,P,S,T |

| Country | Hepatitis A vaccine recommended | Japanese encephalitis vaccine recommended | Japanese encephalitis endemic areas | Poliomyelitis vaccine recommended | Typhoid vaccine recommended | Typhoid vaccine recommended for some travellers | Yellow fever — Vaccine required | Yellow fever — Vaccine recommended for some travellers | Yellow fever — Vaccine required if travelling from certain areas | Malaria — Malarious areas present | Malaria — Chloroquine resistance | Rabies-free or not recently reported | Tick-borne encephalitis present in some areas | Other endemic diseases |
|---|---|---|---|---|---|---|---|---|---|---|---|---|---|---|
| British Virgin Islands | ✓ | | | | | | | | | | | ✓ | | |
| Brunei Darussalam | ✓ | ✓ | | ✓ | ✓ | | | | ✓ | | | ✓ | | D,Fa,F,Pa |
| Bulgaria | ✓ | | | ✓ | ✓ | | | | | | | | ✓ | |
| Burkina Faso | ✓ | | | ✓ | ✓ | ✓ | ✓ | | | ✓ | ✓ | | | F,H,O,S,T |
| Burundi | ✓ | | | ✓ | ✓ | ✓ | | ✓ | ✓ | ✓ | ✓ | | | F,H,S,T,Ti |
| Cambodia | ✓ | | ✓ | ✓ | ✓ | | | | ✓ | ✓ | ✓ | | | D,Fa,F,Pa |
| Cameroon | ✓ | | | ✓ | ✓ | ✓ | ✓ | | | ✓ | ✓ | | | D,F,H,O,Pa,S,T,Ti |
| Canada | | | | | | | | | | | | | | |
| Cape Verde | ✓ | | | ✓ | ✓ | | | | ✓ | ✓ | | ✓ | | D,F,H,L,Ti |
| Cayman Islands | ✓ | | | | | | | | | | | ✓ | | |
| Central African Republic | ✓ | | | ✓ | ✓ | ✓ | ✓ | | | ✓ | ✓ | | | F,H,O,S,T |
| Chad | ✓ | | | ✓ | ✓ | ✓ | | ✓ | ✓ | ✓ | ✓ | | | F,H,O,S,T,Ti |
| Chile | ✓ | | | | ✓ | | | | | | | | | T |
| China | ✓ | ✓ | ✓ | | ✓ | ✓ | | | ✓ | ✓ | ✓ | | | C,D,Fa,F,H,L,P,Pa,S |
| Christmas Island | | | | | | ✓ | ✓ | | | | | | | |
| Colombia | | | | | ✓ | | | ✓ | | ✓ | ✓ | | | D,L,O,T |
| Comoros | ✓ | | | ✓ | ✓ | | | | | ✓ | ✓ | | | D,F,H,L,O |
| Congo | ✓ | | | ✓ | ✓ | | ✓ | | | ✓ | ✓ | | | F,H,O,P,S,T |

| | Hepatitis A vaccine recommended | Japanese encephalitis vaccine recommended | Japanese encephalitis endemic areas | Poliomyelitis vaccine recommended | Typhoid vaccine recommended | Typhoid vaccine recommended for some travellers | Yellow fever — Vaccine required | Yellow fever — Vaccine recommended for some travellers | Yellow fever — Vaccine required if travelling from certain areas | Malaria — Malarious areas present | Malaria — Chloroquine resistance | Rabies-free or not recently reported | Tick-borne encephalitis present in some areas | Other endemic diseases |
|---|---|---|---|---|---|---|---|---|---|---|---|---|---|---|
| Cook Islands | ✓ | | | ✓ | ✓ | | | | | | | ✓ | | D,F |
| Costa Rica | ✓ | | | ✓ | ✓ | | | | | ✓ | | | | D,F,L,T |
| Cote d'Ivoire | ✓ | | ✓ | ✓ | ✓ | ✓ | ✓ | | | ✓ | ✓ | | | F,H,O,S,T |
| Croatia | ✓ | | | | ✓ | | | | | | | | | |
| Cuba | ✓ | | | | ✓ | | | | | | | ✓ | | D |
| Cyprus | ✓ | | | ✓ | ✓ | | | | | | | | | |
| Czech Republic | | | | | | | | | | | | | ✓ | |
| Democratic Republic of Congo (Zaire) | ✓ | | ✓ | ✓ | ✓ | ✓ | ✓ | | | ✓ | ✓ | | | F,H,L,O,S,T |
| Denmark | | | | | | | | | | | | ✓ | | |
| Djibouti | ✓ | | | ✓ | ✓ | ✓ | | | ✓ | ✓ | ✓ | | | F,H,S |
| Dominica | ✓ | | | | ✓ | | | | ✓ | | | | | D |
| Dominican Republic | ✓ | | | | ✓ | | | | ✓ | ✓ | | | | D,L,S |
| Ecuador | ✓ | | | | ✓ | ✓ | | ✓ | ✓ | ✓ | ✓ | | | D,O,P,Pa,T |
| Egypt | ✓ | | | ✓ | ✓ | | | | ✓ | ✓ | | | | |
| El Salvador | ✓ | | | ✓ | ✓ | | | | ✓ | ✓ | | | | D,L,T |
| Equatorial Guinea | ✓ | | | ✓ | ✓ | | | ✓ | ✓ | ✓ | ✓ | | | H,L,O,Pa,S |
| Eritrea | ✓ | | | | ✓ | | | | | ✓ | ✓ | | | |

| | Hepatitis A vaccine recommended | Japanese encephalitis vaccine recommended | Japanese encephalitis endemic areas | Poliomyelitis vaccine recommended | Typhoid vaccine recommended | Typhoid vaccine recommended for some travellers | Yellow fever: Vaccine required | Yellow fever: Vaccine recommended for some travellers | Yellow fever: Vaccine required if travelling from certain areas | Malaria: Malarious areas present | Malaria: Chloroquine resistance | Rabies-free or not recently reported | Tick-borne encephalitis present in some areas | Other endemic diseases |
|---|---|---|---|---|---|---|---|---|---|---|---|---|---|---|
| Estonia | ✓ | | | | | | | | | | | | | |
| Ethiopia | ✓ | | | ✓ | ✓ | ✓ | | ✓ | ✓ | ✓ | ✓ | | | H,L,O,S |
| Falkland Islands | | | | | | | | | | | | | | |
| Faroe Islands | | | | | | | | | | | | ✓ | | |
| Fiji | ✓ | | | | ✓ | | | | ✓ | | | ✓ | | D,F |
| Finland | | | | | | | | | | | | ✓ | ✓ | |
| France | | | | | | | | | | | | | | L |
| French Guiana | ✓ | | | ✓ | ✓ | ✓ | ✓ | | ✓ | ✓ | ✓ | | | D,F,S,T |
| French Polynesia | ✓ | | | ✓ | ✓ | | ✓ | | | | | ✓ | | D,F |
| Gabon | ✓ | | | ✓ | ✓ | ✓ | | ✓ | | ✓ | ✓ | | | F,H,O,Pa,S |
| Gambia | ✓ | | | ✓ | ✓ | ✓ | | | ✓ | ✓ | ✓ | | | F,H,O,S,T |
| Georgia | ✓ | | | | ✓ | | | | | | | | | |
| Germany | | | | | | | | | | | | | ✓ | |
| Ghana | ✓ | | | ✓ | ✓ | ✓ | ✓ | | ✓ | ✓ | ✓ | | | F,H,O,S,T |
| Gibraltar | | | | | | | | | | | | ✓ | | |
| Greece | | | | | | | | | | | | ✓ | | L |
| Greenland | | | | | | | | | | | | | | |
| Grenada | | | | | | | | | | | | | | D |

135

| Country | Hepatitis A vaccine recommended | Japanese encephalitis vaccine recommended | Japanese encephalitis endemic areas | Poliomyelitis vaccine recommended | Typhoid vaccine recommended | Typhoid vaccine recommended for some travellers | Yellow fever – Vaccine required | Yellow fever – Vaccine recommended for some travellers | Yellow fever – Vaccine required if travelling from certain areas | Malaria – Malarious areas present | Malaria – Chloroquine resistance | Rabies-free or not recently reported | Tick-borne encephalitis present in some areas | Other endemic diseases |
|---|---|---|---|---|---|---|---|---|---|---|---|---|---|---|
| Guadeloupe | ✓ | | | | | | | | ✓ | | | ✓ | | D,S |
| Guam | ✓ | | | ✓ | ✓ | | | | | | | ✓ | | D,F |
| Guatemala | ✓ | | ✓ | | ✓ | | | | ✓ | | | | | D,O |
| Guinea | ✓ | | ✓ | ✓ | | ✓ | | ✓ | ✓ | ✓ | ✓ | | | D,H,O,S,T |
| Guinea-Bissau | ✓ | | | ✓ | | ✓ | | ✓ | ✓ | ✓ | ✓ | | | F,H,O,S,T |
| Guyana | ✓ | | | | | ✓ | | ✓ | ✓ | ✓ | ✓ | | | D,F,S,T |
| Haiti | ✓ | | | | ✓ | | | | ✓ | ✓ | | | | D,F |
| Honduras | | | | | | | | | ✓ | ✓ | | | | D,F |
| Hong Kong | | | | | | | | | | | | ✓ | | |
| Hungary | | | | | | | | | | | | | ✓ | |
| Iceland | | | | | | | | | | | | ✓ | | |
| India | ✓ | ✓ | ✓ | ✓ | ✓ | | | | ✓ | ✓ | ✓ | | | D,F,H,I,P |
| Indonesia | ✓ | ✓ | | ✓ | ✓ | | | | ✓ | ✓ | ✓ | | | D,Fa,F,Pa |
| Iran | ✓ | | | ✓ | ✓ | | | | ✓ | ✓ | ✓ | | | H |
| Iraq | ✓ | | | ✓ | ✓ | | | | ✓ | ✓ | | ✓ | | H,L,S |
| Ireland | | | | | | | | | | | | | | |
| Israel | ✓ | | | ✓ | | | | | | | | | | |
| Italy | | | | | | | | | | | | ✓ | | L |

| Country | Hepatitis A vaccine recommended | Japanese encephalitis vaccine recommended | Japanese encephalitis endemic areas | Poliomyelitis vaccine recommended | Typhoid vaccine recommended | Typhoid vaccine recommended for some travellers | Yellow fever: Vaccine required | Yellow fever: Vaccine recommended for some travellers | Yellow fever: Vaccine required if travelling from certain areas | Malaria: Malarious areas present | Malaria: Chloroquine resistance | Rabies-free or not recently reported | Tick-borne encephalitis present in some areas | Other endemic diseases |
|---|---|---|---|---|---|---|---|---|---|---|---|---|---|---|
| Jamaica | ✓ | | | | ✓ | | | | ✓ | | | ✓ | | D |
| Japan | | ✓ | | | | | | | | | | ✓ | | C,S,Pa |
| Jordan | ✓ | | | ✓ | ✓ | | | | ✓ | | | | | |
| Kazakhstan | ✓ | | ✓ | ✓ | ✓ | | | | ✓ | | | | | |
| Kenya | ✓ | | | ✓ | | ✓ | | ✓ | ✓ | ✓ | ✓ | | | D,F,H,I,P,S |
| Kiribat | ✓ | | | ✓ | ✓ | | | | ✓ | | | ✓ | | D,F |
| Korea, North | ✓ | ✓ | | | ✓ | | | | | | | | | C,D,F,H,Pa |
| Korea, South | ✓ | ✓ | | ✓ | ✓ | | | | | ✓ | | | | |
| Kuwait | ✓ | | | | ✓ | | | | | | | | | |
| Kyrgyzstan | ✓ | | | | ✓ | | | | | | | | | |
| Laos | ✓ | ✓ | | ✓ | | ✓ | ✓ | | | ✓ | ✓ | ✓ | | D,F,Pa |
| Latvia | | | | | | | | | | | | | | |
| Lebancn | ✓ | | | ✓ | ✓ | | | | ✓ | | | | | |
| Lesotho | ✓ | | | ✓ | ✓ | | | | ✓ | | | | | S |
| Liberia | ✓ | | | ✓ | ✓ | | | | ✓ | ✓ | ✓ | | | H |
| Libya | ✓ | | | | ✓ | | | | | ✓ | | ✓ | | F,H,O,Pa,S,T |
| Liechtenstein | | | | | | | | | | | | | | |
| Lithuania | ✓ | | | | ✓ | | | | | | | | | |

| Country | Hepatitis A vaccine recommended | Japanese encephalitis vaccine recommended | Japanese encephalitis endemic areas | Poliomyelitis vaccine recommended | Typhoid vaccine recommended | Typhoid vaccine recommended for some travellers | Yellow fever: Vaccine required | Yellow fever: Vaccine recommended for some travellers | Yellow fever: Vaccine required if travelling from certain areas | Malaria: Malarious areas present | Malaria: Chloroquine resistance | Rabies-free or not recently reported | Tick-borne encephalitis present in some areas | Other endemic diseases |
|---|---|---|---|---|---|---|---|---|---|---|---|---|---|---|
| Luxembourg |  |  |  |  | ✓ |  |  |  |  |  |  |  |  |  |
| Macao | ✓ |  |  | ✓ | ✓ |  |  |  |  |  |  | ✓ |  | C,D,H,Pa |
| Macedonia | ✓ |  |  |  | ✓ |  |  |  |  |  |  |  |  |  |
| Madagascar | ✓ |  |  | ✓ | ✓ |  |  |  | ✓ | ✓ | ✓ |  |  | F,H,P,S,Ti |
| Malawi | ✓ |  |  | ✓ | ✓ |  |  |  | ✓ | ✓ | ✓ |  |  | F,H,O,S,T,Ti |
| Malaysia | ✓ | ✓ |  | ✓ | ✓ |  |  |  | ✓ | ✓ | ✓ |  |  | D,Fa,F |
| Maldives | ✓ |  |  | ✓ | ✓ |  |  |  | ✓ | ✓ | ✓ |  |  | D,F |
| Mali | ✓ |  | ✓ | ✓ | ✓ | ✓ | ✓ |  | ✓ | ✓ | ✓ | ✓ |  | F,H,O,S,T,Ti |
| Malta |  |  |  |  |  |  |  |  |  |  |  | ✓ |  | L |
| Marshall Islands | ✓ |  |  |  | ✓ |  |  |  |  |  |  | ✓ |  |  |
| Martinique | ✓ |  |  |  | ✓ |  |  |  | ✓ | ✓ | ✓ | ✓ |  | D,S |
| Mauritania | ✓ |  |  | ✓ | ✓ |  | ✓ |  |  | ✓ | ✓ |  |  | F,H,L,O,S,Ti |
| Mauritius | ✓ |  |  | ✓ | ✓ |  |  |  | ✓ | ✓ |  | ✓ |  |  |
| Mayotte | ✓ |  | ✓ | ✓ | ✓ |  |  |  | ✓ | ✓ |  |  |  | D,F,L,O |
| Mexico | ✓ |  |  |  | ✓ |  |  |  |  |  |  |  |  | D,L,O,T |
| Moldova | ✓ |  |  |  | ✓ |  |  |  |  |  |  |  |  |  |
| Monaco |  |  |  |  |  |  |  |  |  |  |  | ✓ |  |  |
| Mongolia | ✓ |  |  | ✓ | ✓ |  |  |  |  |  |  |  |  | D,P |

138

| Country | Hepatitis A vaccine recommended | Japanese encephalitis vaccine recommended | Japanese encephalitis endemic areas | Poliomyelitis vaccine recommended | Typhoid vaccine recommended | Typhoid vaccine recommended for some travellers | Yellow fever: Vaccine required | Yellow fever: Vaccine recommended for some travellers | Yellow fever: Vaccine required if travelling from certain areas | Malaria: Malarious areas present | Malaria: Chloroquine resistance | Rabies-free or not recently reported | Tick-borne encephalitis present in some areas | Other endemic diseases |
|---|---|---|---|---|---|---|---|---|---|---|---|---|---|---|
| Montserrat | ✓ | | | | ✓ | | | | | | | | | D |
| Morocco | ✓ | | | ✓ | ✓ | | | | | | | | | S |
| Mozambique | ✓ | ✓ | | ✓ | ✓ | | | | ✓ | ✓ | ✓ | | | F,H,P,S,T,Ti |
| Myanmar | ✓ | | | ✓ | ✓ | | | | ✓ | ✓ | ✓ | | | D,F,P,Pa |
| Namibia | ✓ | | | ✓ | ✓ | | | | ✓ | ✓ | ✓ | | | H,S,T |
| Nauru | ✓ | | | | ✓ | | | | ✓ | | | | | D,F |
| Nepal | ✓ | ✓ | ✓ | ✓ | ✓ | | | | ✓ | ✓ | ✓ | | | D,L |
| Netherlands | | | | | | | | | | | | | | |
| Netherlands Antilles | ✓ | | | ✓ | ✓ | | | ✓ | | | | | | |
| New Caledonia | ✓ | | | ✓ | ✓ | | | ✓ | ✓ | | | ✓ | | D,F |
| New Zealand | | | | | | | | | | | | ✓ | | |
| Nicaragua | ✓ | | | ✓ | ✓ | | | | ✓ | | | | | D,L,T |
| Niger | ✓ | | ✓ | ✓ | ✓ | ✓ | | | ✓ | ✓ | ✓ | ✓ | | F,H,O,S,T,Ti |
| Nigeria | ✓ | | ✓ | ✓ | ✓ | ✓ | | | ✓ | ✓ | ✓ | | | D,F,H,O,S,T |
| Niue Island | ✓ | | | ✓ | ✓ | | | | | | | ✓ | | D,F,S |
| Northern Mariana Islands | ✓ | | | ✓ | | | | | | | | | | D,F |
| Norway | | | | | | | | | | | | ✓ | ✓ | |
| Oman | ✓ | | | ✓ | ✓ | | | | ✓ | ✓ | ✓ | | | F,S |

| Country | Hepatitis A vaccine recommended | Japanese encephalitis vaccine recommended | Japanese encephalitis endemic areas | Poliomyelitis vaccine recommended | Typhoid vaccine recommended | Typhoid vaccine recommended for some travellers | Yellow fever: Vaccine required | Yellow fever: Vaccine recommended for some travellers | Yellow fever: Vaccine required if travelling from certain areas | Malaria: Malarious areas present | Malaria: Chloroquine resistance | Rabies-free or not recently reported | Tick-borne encephalitis present in some areas | Other endemic diseases |
|---|---|---|---|---|---|---|---|---|---|---|---|---|---|---|
| Pakistan | ✓ | ✓ | | ✓ | ✓ | | | | ✓ | ✓ | ✓ | | | D,H,L |
| Palau | ✓ | | | | ✓ | | | | | | | | | |
| Panama | ✓ | | | | ✓ | ✓ | | ✓ | | ✓ | ✓ | | | D |
| Papua New Guinea | ✓ | ✓ | | ✓ | ✓ | | | | ✓ | ✓ | ✓ | ✓ | | D,F |
| Paraguay | ✓ | | | | ✓ | | | ✓ | ✓ | ✓ | | | | L,T |
| Peru | ✓ | ✓ | | ✓ | ✓ | ✓ | | ✓ | ✓ | ✓ | ✓ | | | L,P,Pa,T |
| Philippines | ✓ | | | ✓ | ✓ | | | | ✓ | ✓ | ✓ | | | D,Fa,F,Pa,S |
| Pitcairn | ✓ | | ✓ | ✓ | | | | | | | | | | D |
| Poland | ✓ | | | | ✓ | | | | | | | | ✓ | |
| Portugal | ✓ | | | | | | | | | | | ✓ | | L,S |
| Puerto Rico | ✓ | | | ✓ | ✓ | | | | | | | | | |
| Qatar | ✓ | | | ✓ | ✓ | | | | | | | | | |
| Reunion Island | ✓ | | | ✓ | ✓ | | | | ✓ | | | ✓ | | |
| Romania | ✓ | | | ✓ | ✓ | | | | | | | ✓ | | |
| Russian Federation | ✓ | ✓ | | ✓ | ✓ | | | | | | | | ✓ | H,L |
| Rwanda | ✓ | | | | ✓ | ✓ | ✓ | | ✓ | ✓ | ✓ | | ✓ | F,H,O,P,S,T,Ti |
| Saint Helena | ✓ | | | | ✓ | | | | ✓ | | | | | D |
| Saint Kitts and Nevis | ✓ | | | | ✓ | | | | | | | ✓ | | D |

| | Hepatitis A vaccine recommended | Japanese encephalitis vaccine recommended | Japanese encephalitis endemic areas | Poliomyelitis vaccine recommended | Typhoid vaccine recommended | Typhoid vaccine recommended for some travellers | Yellow fever: Vaccine required | Yellow fever: Vaccine recommended for some travellers | Yellow fever: Vaccine required if travelling from certain areas | Malaria: Malarious areas present | Malaria: Chloroquine resistance | Rabies-free or not recently reported | Tick-borne encephalitis present in some areas | Other endemic diseases |
|---|---|---|---|---|---|---|---|---|---|---|---|---|---|---|
| Saint Lucia | ✓ | | | | ✓ | | | | ✓ | | | | | D |
| Saint Pierre and Miquelon | ✓ | | | | ✓ | | | | | | | ✓ | | D |
| Saint Vincent | ✓ | | | ✓ | ✓ | | | | ✓ | | | ✓ | | D,F |
| Samoa | ✓ | | | ✓ | ✓ | | | | ✓ | | | | | D,F |
| San Marino | | | | | | | ✓ | | | | | | | |
| Sao Tome and Principe | ✓ | | ✓ | ✓ | ✓ | ✓ | | | ✓ | ✓ | ✓ | | | F,H,S |
| Saudi Arabia | ✓ | | | ✓ | ✓ | | | ✓ | | ✓ | ✓ | | | L,S |
| Senegal | ✓ | | ✓ | ✓ | ✓ | ✓ | | | ✓ | ✓ | ✓ | | | F,H,O,S,T,Ti |
| Serbia/Montenegro | ✓ | | | | ✓ | | | | | | | | | |
| Seychelles | ✓ | | | ✓ | ✓ | | | | ✓ | | | ✓ | | |
| Sierra Leone | ✓ | | ✓ | ✓ | ✓ | ✓ | | ✓ | ✓ | ✓ | ✓ | | | F,H,O,S,T,Ti |
| Singapore | | | | | ✓ | ✓ | | | ✓ | | | ✓ | | D |
| Slovakia | | | | | ✓ | | | | | | | | | |
| Slovenia | ✓ | | | | ✓ | | | | | | | | | |
| Solomon Islands | ✓ | | | ✓ | ✓ | | | | ✓ | ✓ | ✓ | ✓ | | D,F |
| Somalia | ✓ | | | ✓ | ✓ | | | | ✓ | ✓ | ✓ | | | D,F,H,S |
| South Africa | ✓ | | | ✓ | ✓ | | | | ✓ | ✓ | ✓ | | | H,S |
| Spain | | | | | | | | | | | | ✓ | | L |

| Country | Hepatitis A vaccine recommended | Japanese encephalitis vaccine recommended | Japanese encephalitis endemic areas | Poliomyelitis vaccine recommended | Typhoid vaccine recommended | Typhoid vaccine recommended for some travellers | Yellow fever: Vaccine required | Yellow fever: Vaccine recommended for some travellers | Yellow fever: Vaccine required if travelling from certain areas | Malaria: Malarious areas present | Malaria: Chloroquine resistance | Rabies-free or not recently reported | Tick-borne encephalitis present in some areas | Other endemic diseases |
|---|---|---|---|---|---|---|---|---|---|---|---|---|---|---|
| Sri Lanka | ✓ | ✓ | | ✓ | ✓ | | | | ✓ | ✓ | ✓ | | | D,F |
| Sudan | ✓ | | ✓ | ✓ | ✓ | ✓ | | ✓ | ✓ | ✓ | ✓ | | | F,H,I,O,S,T,Ti |
| Suriname | ✓ | | | ✓ | ✓ | ✓ | | ✓ | ✓ | ✓ | ✓ | | | D,L,F,H,S,T |
| Swaziland | ✓ | | ✓ | ✓ | ✓ | | | | ✓ | ✓ | ✓ | | | H,S |
| Sweden | | | | | | | | | | | | ✓ | ✓ | |
| Switzerland | | | | | | | | | | | | | ✓ | |
| Syria | ✓ | | | ✓ | ✓ | | | | ✓ | ✓ | | | | L,S,Ti |
| Taiwan | ✓ | | | | ✓ | | | | ✓ | | | ✓ | | |
| Tajikistan | ✓ | | | | ✓ | | | | | ✓ | ? | | | |
| Tanzania | ✓ | | ✓ | ✓ | ✓ | ✓ | | ✓ | ✓ | ✓ | ✓ | | | F,H,O,P,S,T |
| Thailand | ✓ | ✓ | | ✓ | ✓ | ✓ | | | ✓ | ✓ | ✓ | | | D,Fa,Fpa |
| Togo | ✓ | | | ✓ | ✓ | | ✓ | | ✓ | ✓ | ✓ | | | F,H,O,S,T,Ti |
| Tonga | ✓ | | | ✓ | | | | | ✓ | | | ✓ | | D,F |
| Trinidad and Tobago | ✓ | | | ✓ | ✓ | | | | ✓ | | | | | D |
| Tunisia | ✓ | | | ✓ | ✓ | | | | | | | | | L,S |
| Turkey | ✓ | | | ✓ | ✓ | | | | | ✓ | | | | L,Ti |
| Turkmenistan | ✓ | | | | ✓ | | | | | | | | | |
| Tuvalu | ✓ | | | ✓ | ✓ | | | | | | | | | D,F |

| Country | Hepatitis A vaccine recommended | Japanese encephalitis vaccine recommended | Japanese encephalitis endemic areas | Poliomyelitis vaccine recommended | Typhoid vaccine recommended | Typhoid vaccine recommended for some travellers | Yellow fever — Vaccine required | Yellow fever — Vaccine recommended for some travellers | Yellow fever — Vaccine required if travelling from certain areas | Malaria — Malarious areas present | Malaria — Chloroquine resistance | Rabies-free or not recently reported | Tick-borne encephalitis present in some areas | Other endemic diseases |
|---|---|---|---|---|---|---|---|---|---|---|---|---|---|---|
| Uganda | ✓ | | ✓ | ✓ | ✓ | ✓ | | ✓ | ✓ | ✓ | ✓ | | | F,H,O,P,S,T,Ti |
| Ukraine | ✓ | | | | ✓ | | | | | | | | | |
| United Arab Emirates | ✓ | | | ✓ | ✓ | | | | | ✓ | ✓ | | | L,Ti |
| United Kingdom | | | | | | | | | | | | ✓ | | |
| US of America | | | | | | | | | | | | | | |
| Uruguay | ✓ | | | | ✓ | | | | | | | ✓ | | T |
| Uzbekistan | ✓ | | | | ✓ | | | | | | | | | |
| Vanuatu | ✓ | | | ✓ | ✓ | | | | | ✓ | ✓ | ✓ | | D,F |
| Venezuela | ✓ | | | | ✓ | ✓ | | ✓ | | ✓ | ✓ | | | D,O,Pa,S,T |
| Vietnam | ✓ | ✓ | | ✓ | ✓ | | | | ✓ | ✓ | ✓ | | | D,Fa,F,P,Pa |
| Virgin Islands (USA) | | | | | | | | | | | | ✓ | | |
| Yemen | ✓ | | | ✓ | ✓ | ✓ | | | ✓ | ✓ | ✓ | | | Dr,L,O,S |
| Zambia | ✓ | | ✓ | ✓ | ✓ | | | ✓ | | ✓ | ✓ | | | F,H,S,T |
| Zimbabwe | ✓ | | | ✓ | ✓ | | | | | ✓ | ✓ | | | F,H,P,S |

# Key references

## GENERAL

Auerbach PS, ed. *Wilderness Medicine.* 3rd edn. St Louis: Mosby, 1995.

Cook GC. *Travel-associated Disease.* London: Royal College of Physicians, 1995.

Cook GC, ed. *Manson's Tropical Diseases.* 20th edn. London: WB Saunders, 1996.

DuPont HL, Steffen R, eds. *Textbook of Travel Medicine and Health.* Hamilton, Ontario: Decker, 1997.

Jong E, McMullen R. *The Travel and Tropical Medicine Manual.* 2nd edn. Philadelphia: WB Saunders, 1995.

Schlossberg D, ed. *Infections of Leisure.* 2nd edn. Washington, DC: American Society for Microbiology, 1999.

Steedman DJ. *Environmental Medical Emergencies.* Oxford: Oxford University Press, 1994.

Strickland GT, ed. *Hunter's Tropical Medicine and Emerging Infectious Diseases.* 8th edn. Philadelphia, PA: WB Saunders, 2000.

Walker E, Williams G, Raeside F. *ABC of Healthy Travel.* London: BMJ Publishing Group, 1993.

Warrell D, Anderson S. *Expedition Medicine. Royal Geographical Society.* London: Profile Books, 1998.

Wilson ME. *A World Guide to Infections: Diseases, Distribution, Diagnosis.* New York: Oxford University Press, 1991.

## INDIVIDUALS WITH SPECIAL CONSIDERATIONS

Benson E, Metz R. Management of diabetes during intercontinental travel. *Bull Mason Clinic* 1984–1985;38:145–51.

Centers for Disease Control and Prevention. *Health Information for International Travel 1999–2000.* Atlanta, GA: DHHS, 1999.

Dessery BL, Robin MR, Pasini W. The aged, infirm, or handicapped traveler. In: DuPont HL, Steffen R, eds. *Textbook of Travel Medicine and Health.* Hamilton, Ontario: Decker, 1997:320–8.

Karp CL, Neva FA. Tropical infectious diseases in human immunodeficiency virus-infected patients. *Clin Infect Dis* 1999;28:947–65.

Phillips-Howard PA, Steffen R, Kerr L *et al.* Safety of mefloquine and other antimalarial agents in the first trimester of pregnancy. *J Travel Med* 1998;5:121–6.

Simons FMJ, Cobelens FGJ, Danner SA. Common health problems in HIV-infected travelers to the (sub)tropics. *J Travel Med* 1999;6:71–5.

Van Gompel A, Kozarsky P, Colebunders R. Adult travelers with HIV infection. *J Travel Med* 1997;4:136–43.

## MOTION SICKNESS AND JET LAG

Avery D, Lenz M, Landis C. Guidelines for prescribing melatonin. *Ann Med* 1998; 30:122–30.

McIntosh IB. Motion sickness – questions and answers. *J Travel Med* 1998;5:89–91.

Nicholson AN, Pascoe PA, Spencer MB, Benson AJ. Jet lag and motion sickness. *Br Med Bull* 1993;49:285–304.

Oosterveld W. Motion sickness. *J Travel Med* 1995;2:182–5.

Petrie KJ, Dawson AG. Recent developments in the treatment of jet lag. *J Travel Med* 1994;1:79–83.

Schmid R, Schick T, Steffen R *et al.* Comparison of seven commonly used agents for prophylaxis of seasickness. *J Travel Med* 1994;1:203–6.

Waterhouse J, Reilly T, Atkinson G. Jet-lag. *Lancet* 1997;350:1611–16.

## VACCINES

*Canadian Immunizations Guide, Fifth Edition.* Minister of Public Works and Government Services Canada, 1998.

Jong EC. Travel immunizations. *Med Clin N Am* 1999;83:903–22.

Pollard AJ, Levin M. Vaccines for prevention of meningococcal disease. *Ped Infect Dis J* 2000;19:333–45.

Salisbury DM, Begg N. *Immunization against Infectious Diseases.* London: HMSO, 1996.

The Yellow book (www.cdc.gov/travel/hcwvax.htm)

Thompson RF, Bass DM, Hoffman SL. Travel vaccines. *Infect Dis Clin N Am* 1999;13:149–67.

## MALARIA

Baird JK, Hoffman SL. Prevention of malaria in travellers. *Med Clin N Am* 1999;83:923–43.

Collins WE, Jeffery GM. Primaquine resistance in *Plasmodium vivax. Am J Trop Med Hyg* 1996;55:243–9.

Holder AA. Malaria vaccines. *Proc Natl Acad Sci USA* 1999;96:1167–9.

Jelinek T, Amsler L, Grobusch MP, Nothdurft HD. Self-use of rapid tests for malaria diagnosis by tourists. *Lancet* 1999;354:1609.

Longworth DL. Drug-resistant malaria in children and travellers. *Ped Clin N Am* 1995;42:649–65.

Newton P, White N. Malaria: new developments in treatment and prevention. *Annu Rev Med* 1999;50:179–92.

White NJ. Drug resistance in malaria. *Br Med Bull* 1998;54:703–15.

## OTHER DISEASES TRANSMITTED BY MOSQUITOES

Rigau-Perez JG, Clark GG, Gubler DJ *et al.* Dengue and dengue haemorrhagic fever. *Lancet* 1998;352:971–7.

Thisyakorn U, Thisyakorn C, Wilde H. Japanese encephalitis and international travel. *J Travel Med* 1995;2:37–40.

Tsai TR, Chang GW, Yu YX. Japanese encephalitis vaccines. In: Plotkin SA, Orenstein WA, eds. *Vaccines.* 3rd edn. Philadelphia, PA: WB Saunders, 1999:672–710.

WHO. *Dengue Haemorrhagic Fever: Diagnosis, Treatment, Prevention and Control.* 2nd edn. Geneva: WHO, 1997.

WHO. *District Guidelines for Yellow Fever Surveillance.* Geneva: WHO, 1998.

## FOOD- AND WATER-BORNE ILLNESS

Ansdell VE, Ericsson CD. Prevention and empiric treatment of traveller's diarrhea. *Med Clin N Am* 1999;83:945–73.

Backer HD. Field water disinfection. In: Auerbach PA, ed. *Wilderness Medicine: Management of Wilderness and Environmental Emergencies*. St Louis: Mosby Year Book, 1995:1060–110.

Caeiro J-P, DuPont HL. Management of travellers diarrhoea. *Drugs* 1998; 56:73–81.

Forgey WW. *Wilderness Medical Society Practice Guidelines for Wilderness Emergency Care*. Merrillville, IN: ICS Books, 1995.

Kotloff KL. Bacterial diarrheal pathogens. *Adv Ped Infect Dis* 1999;14:219–66.

Morris JG. *Pfiesteria*, "the cell from hell", and other toxic algal nightmares. *Clin Infect Dis* 1999;28:1191–8.

Shlim DR. Travelers' diarrhea. *Wild Environ Med* 1999;10:165–70.

Staat MA. Travellers diarrhea. *Ped Infect Dis J* 1999;18:373–4.

Steele JCH, ed. Food-borne diseases. *Clin Lab Med* 1999;19:469–712.

WHO. Chagas: geographical distribution. www.who.int/ctd/chagas/geo.htm

WHO. Schistosomiasis: epidemiological data/geographical distribution. www.who.int/ctd/schisto/epidemio.htm

WHO. Trypanosomiasis: geographical distribution 1997. www.who.int/emc/diseases/tryp/trypanogeo.html

## OTHER PARASITIC DISEASES

Centers for Disease Control and Prevention. Lyme disease: geographical distribution 1998. www.cdc.gov/ncidod/dvbid/LD_dotden_98.gif

Jelinek T, Nothdurft H-D, Löscher T. Schistosomiasis in travelers and expatriates. *J Travel Med* 1996;3:160–4.

Pearson RD, de Queiroz Sousa A. Clinical spectrum of leishmaniasis. *Clin Infect Dis* 1996;22:1–13.

Ponce-de-Leon S, Lisker-Melman M, Kato-Maeda M et al. *Trypanosoma brucei rhodesiense* infection imported to Mexico from a tourist resort in Kenya. *Clin Infect Dis* 1996;23:847–8.

## DISEASES TRANSMITTED BY TICKS, LICE, MITES AND FLEAS

Centers for Disease Control and Prevention. Health Information for International Travel 1999–2000. DHHS: USA, 1999.

Jacobs RF, Schutze GE. The camper's uninvited guests. In: Schlossberg D, ed. *Infections of Leisure*. 2nd edn. Washington, DC: American Society for Microbiology, 1999:125–43.

Parola P, Vogelaers D, Roure C et al. Murine typhus in travelers returning from Indonesia. *Emerg Infect Dis* 1998; 4:677–80.

Stanek G. Borreliosis and travel medicine. *J Travel Med* 1995;2:244–51.

## MISCELLANEOUS INFECTIOUS DISEASES

Anon. Control and prevention of meningococcal disease: recommendations of the Advisory Committee on Immunization Practices (ACIP). *MMWR Morb Mortal Wkly Rep* 1997;46(RR-5):1–10.

Anon. Meningococcal. In: Salisbury DM, Begg NT, eds. *Immunization against Infectious Disease*. London: HMSO, 1996:147–54.

Antony SJ. Leptospirosis – an emerging pathogen in travel medicine: a review of its clinical manifestations and management. *J Travel Med* 1996;3:113–18.

Dye C, Scheele S, Dolin P et al. Global burden of tuberculosis. Estimated incidence, prevalence, and mortality by country. *JAMA* 1999;282:677–86.

Haupt W. Rabies – risk of exposure and current trends in prevention of human cases. *Vaccine* 1999;17:1742–9.

Hemachudha T, Phuapradit P. Rabies. *Curr Opin Neurol* 1997;10:26–67.

Houston S. Tuberculosis risk and prevention in travelers – what about BCG? *J Travel Med* 1997;4:76–82.

Jones D. Epidemiology of meningococcal disease in Europe and the USA. In: Cartwright K, ed. *Meningococcal Disease*. 1st edn. Chichester: Wiley, 1995:147–57.

Lang J, Plotkin SA. Rabies risk and immunoprophylaxis in children. *Adv Ped Infect Dis* 1998;13:219–55.

Lapeyssonnie L. La meningite cerebrospinale en Afrique. *Bull WHO* 1963;28(Suppl 1):3–114.

Loscher T, Keystone JS, Steffen R. Vaccination of travelers against hepatitis A and B. *J Travel Med* 1999;6:107–14.

Pollard AJ, Britto J, Nadel S et al. Emergency management of meningococcal disease. *Arch Dis Child* 1999;80:290–6.

Wang CC, Celum CL. Global risk of sexually transmitted diseases. *Med Clin N Am* 1999;83:975–95.

Webster RG. Influenza: an emerging disease. *Emerg Infect Dis* 1998;4:436–41.

WHO Expert Committee on Rabies, eighth report. *WHO Tech Rep Ser* 1992;824:1–84. (www.who.int/emc/diseases/zoo/slides/tsld 002.htm)

Zenilman JM. From boudoir to bordello: sexually transmitted diseases and travel. In: Schlossberg D, ed. *Infections of Leisure*. 2nd edn. Washington, DC: American Society for Microbiology, 1999:383–412.

## ENVIRONMENTAL AND CLIMATIC FACTORS

Bewes PC. Trauma and accidents. Practical aspects of the prevention and management of trauma associated with travel. *Br Med Bull* 1993;49:454–64.

Khosla R, Guntupalli KK. Heat-related illness. *Crit Care Clin* 1999;15:251–63.

Kilbourne EM. The spectrum of illness during heat waves. *Am J Prev Med* 1999;16:359–60.

Moon RE. Treatment of diving emergencies. *Crit Care Clin* 1999;15:429–56.

Pollard AJ, Murdoch DR. *The High Altitude Medicine Handbook*. 2nd edn. Oxford: Radcliffe Medical Press, 1998.

Spira A. Diving and marine medicine review. Part I: Diving physics and physiology. *J Travel Med* 1999;6:32–44.

Spira A. Diving and marine medicine review. Part II: Diving diseases. *J Travel Med* 1999;6:180–98.

### RETURNED TRAVELLERS

Kain KC. Skin lesions in returned travellers. *Med Clin N Am* 1999;83:1077–102.

Suh KN, Kozarsky PE, Keystone JS. Evaluation of fever in the returned traveler. *Med Clin N Am* 1999;83:997–1017.

Taylor DN, Connor BA, Shlim DR. Chronic diarrhea in the returned traveler. *Med Clin N Am* 1999;83:1033–54.

Yung AP, Ruff TA. Travel medicine. Upon return. *Med J Aust* 1994;160:206–12.

# Index

acetazolamide 116
Africa
  central 55, 56, 85, 89, 91, 96
  cholera 79
  East 87, 92, 96
  food poisoning 70, 80
  gonorrhoea 106
  loiasis 89
  malaria 41, 42, 45, 46
  North 9, 80, 96
  plague 97
  poliomyelitis 37, 68, 81
  rabies 101, 102
  relapsing fever 96
  returned travellers 128
  schistosomiasis 83, 85
  scorpions 122
  South 94
    poisonous spiders 122
  Southern 10
  spotted fever 94
  sub-Saharan 9, 90, 98, 99, 106
  travellers' diarrhoea 64
  tuberculosis 110
  tungiasis 91
  typhus 92
  West 7, 80, 87, 88, 89
  yellow fever 55, 56
African trypanosomiasis 87–8, 125
aid workers and vaccination 28, 31, 34, 37, 79, 97
air travel 14, 15, 17, 19, 20–1, 25; see also jet lag
altitude sickness 9, 11, 12, 13, 15, 17–18, 115–17
America
  Caribbean 10
    cholera 79, 80
    food poisoning 82
    malaria 46
    rabies-free areas 102
    tungiasis 91
  Latin America 28, 46, 64, 70
  see also Central; North; and South America
ampicillin 67, 77

angiostrongyliasis 68–9, 70–1, 81, 127
Antarctica 13
anthrax 11
arboviral infections 55, 62
  see also Japanese encephalitis
arrhythmias see heart disease
arthropod-borne diseases 9, 10, 13, 62, 68, 70, 81, 84, 92–4
  returned travellers 125
Asia
  food poisoning 72
  Lyme disease 96
  malaria 41
  meningococcal disease 98
  plague 97
  poliomyelitis 37, 68, 81
  rabies 101, 102
  relapsing fever 96
  returned travellers 128
  sexually transmitted infections 106
  spotted fever 94
  travellers' diarrhoea 64
  tuberculosis 109–10
  typhoid 38, 80
  typhus 92
  see also Australasia; East Asia; South-East Asia
Australasia 13
  angiostrongyliasis 68, 81
  cholera 79
  filariasis 88
  food poisoning 72, 82
  Japanese encephalitis 59, 60–1, 62–3
  Lyme disease 96
  meningococcal disease 98
  poisonous spiders 122
  rabies-free areas 102
  sexually transmitted infections 106
  typhus 93, 94
azithromycin 69, 77

benzodiazepines 27
bilharzia see schistosomiasis

blood transfusion
  and Chagas' disease 86
  and hepatitis 127–8
  and malaria 41
  and sexually transmitted infections 107
booster doses 29, 30, 34, 40, 57
  not recommended 38
Borrelia burgdorferi 34
bronchospasm and risk 19
brucellosis 9, 10, 125

Campylobacter 64, 65, 66–7, 77, 80, 124
  vaccine 76
Central America
  angiostrongyliasis 81
  Chagas' disease 86
  food poisoning 70, 72
  malaria 46
  myiasis 90
  onchocerciasis 88–9
  poisonous spiders 122
  schistosomiasis 83
  scorpions 122
  spotted fever 94
  tuberculosis 110
  tungiasis 91
  typhoid 38, 80
  typhus 92
cephalosporins 67, 80, 99, 100
Chagas' disease 10, 11, 86–8
  returned travellers 125
children 7, 15, 17–19
  altitude sickness 17–18
  climate 18–19
  dehydration 77
  dengue 57
  food-borne illness 17, 75–6, 77
  malaria 17, 41
  rabies 101
  travel 15, 17
  typhoid 80
  vaccination 17, 18, 28
  see also meningococcal disease; pertussis; and others by name

chloramphenicol 99, 112
chloroquine 9, 10, 15, 37, 39, 46
  resistance 11, 13, 52, 53, 54,
  131–43
  *see also* malaria,
  chemoprophylaxis
cholera 7, 78–9
  vaccine 16, 22, 28, 30–1, 79
chronic lung disease and risk 19
  *see also* lung disease
ciprofloxacin 78, 80
*Clostridium* 38, 124
co-trimoxazole 67, 69, 78, 79
coeliac disease and risk 36
cold exposure 13, 18, 19, 114–15
*Cryptosporidium* 65, 68–9, 74,
  78, 124
*Culex tritaeniorhyncus* 59

deep vein thrombosis 14
dengue 10, 11, 12, 13
  endemic areas 131–43
  returned travellers 125, 128
diabetes 20, 21, 36
diphtheria vaccination 28–9,
  30–1, 110
diving-related illnesses 118–21
doxycycline 15, 46, 77, 79, 92
  *see also* malaria,
  chemoprophylaxis

East Asia 11
  food poisoning 70
  Japanese encephalitis 59,
  60–1, 62–3
  malaria 46, 52
  spotted fever 94
*Entamoeba histolytica* 65, 68–9,
  78, 124
enteric pathogens 64–5, 66–71,
  124–5, 128 *see also Campylobacter; E. coli; Salmonella; and
  others by name*
eosinophilia
  returned travellers 126–7
*Escherichia coli* 64, 65, 66–7
  vaccine 76
Europe 28, 72, 82, 96,
  102
  Eastern 12, 62–3, 80, 81,
  94–5, 101

Mediterranean 7, 13, 79, 94,
  122
  Western 12–13, 36, 70

fever in returned travellers
  125–6
filariasis 55, 62, 88, 125, 126,
  endemic areas 131–43
fish and shellfish poisoning 10,
  12, 13, 66, 70, 72–3, 78, 81–2
fluke-borne diseases 11, 83–5
food-borne illness 10, 12, 13,
  15, 17, 38, 64–82, 107
  *see also* cholera; travellers'
  diarrhoea; typhoid; *and other
  illnesses by name*
frostbite 115

gamma globulin
  for hepatitis A 29
  *see also* immunoglobulin
*Giardia lamblia* 64–5, 68–9, 74,
  78, 124
gonorrhoea 7, 106

haemorrhagic fever 11
healthcare workers and
  vaccination 31, 34, 37, 97,
  108, 110
heart disease and risk 36
heat-related illness 18, 111–14
hepatitis A 7, 9, 10, 11, 12, 13,
  81, 107, 108
  returned travellers 125, 127–8
  vaccination 18, 29, 30, 31,
  107, 131–43
hepatitis B 9, 10, 12, 106, 107,
  108, 109
  returned travellers 127–8
  vaccination 18, 30, 31, 34,
  107
hepatitis C 107, 108
hepatitis E 9, 12, 81, 108–9
  returned travellers 125, 127–8
  vaccination 16, 18, 22
high-risk groups 5, 7–8, 34
histoplasmosis 10
HIV infection 7, 9, 10, 21, 106
  acute, in returned travellers
  125, 128
  and risk 36, 89

vaccinations for sufferers
  22–3, 29
hyatid disease 9
hypertension and risk 19
hyposplenism 36, 98
hypothermia 114–15

immunoglobulin 29, 30, 37,
  39, 107; *see also* gamma
  globulin
immunosuppression
  and vaccination 31, 33
  increased risk as a result of 7,
  36, 37
Indian subcontinent 12
  cholera 79
  Japanese encephalitis 59,
  60–1, 62–3
  malaria 42, 46, 52
  meningococcal disease 98
  rabies 101
  relapsing fever 96
  schistosomiasis 83
  scorpions 122
  yellow fever 39, 55
infectious diseases *see*
  diphtheria; influenza;
  meningococcal disease; *and
  others by name*
influenza
  returned travellers 125
  vaccination 18, 29, 30–1, 34,
  110
insect-borne diseases 11; *see
  also* malaria; mosquito-borne
  diseases; *and others by name*
insurance 5, 8
intestinal fluke infections 11
intestinal helminth infections 9,
  90, 124, 126–7

Japanese encephalitis 11, 12, 13,
  58, 59, 60–2
  returned travellers 123
  vaccine 16, 18, 22, 30, 31, 34,
  59, 131–43
jaundice
  returned travellers 127–8
jet lag 25–7

*Legionella* infection 7, 125

leishmaniasis 9, 10, 11, 12, 13, 89–90, 131–43
    returned travellers 125
leptospirosis 109, 125, 128
listeriosis 15, 66–7
liver disease and risk 36
loiasis 89, 127
loperamide 77, 78
louse-borne diseases
    relapsing fever 9, 96
    typhus 11, 92
lung disease and risk 36
    see also chronic lung disease
Lyme disease 10, 12, 13, 96–7
    vaccination 18, 30, 31, 34–5

malaria 7, 9, 10, 11, 12, 13, 41–54
    Anopheles 41, 42, 45
    clinical features 43–4
    diagnosis 44
    emergency self-treatment (EST) 49–52
        doses 50, 51, 52
    epidemiology 41–2
    prevention 44–54
        chemoprophylaxis 44, 45–9
            chloroquine 42, 45, 46, 47, 48, 50, 52, 53
            doxycycline 45, 46, 47, 48, 53
            mefloquine 42, 45, 46–8, 51, 53
            proguanil 45, 47, 48, 52
            side-effects 46, 47–8
    returned travellers 125, 126, 128
    risk areas 41, 46, 131–43
    treatment 52–4
    vaccines 49, 131–43
    see also chloroquine; doxycycline; mefloquine; proguanil
measles vaccination 18, 30, 31
measles, mumps and rubella see MMR
mefloquine 11, 15, 39, 46
    see also malaria, chemoprophylaxis
melatonin 26–7
meningococcal disease 7, 9, 12,

98–101
    vaccine 16, 18, 22, 32–3, 35–6, 100–1
metronidazole 69, 71, 78
Middle East 12
    cholera 79
    malaria 46
    meningococcal disease 98, 100–1
    poliomyelitis 81
    relapsing fever 96
    schistosomiasis 83
    scorpions 122
    travellers' diarrhoea 64, 68
MMR vaccination 18, 30, 31, 36
mosquito-borne diseases 55–63
    see also dengue; Japanese encephalitis; malaria; yellow fever
motion sickness 17, 24–5
motor-vehicle accidents 6, 111
myiasis 90

needle sharing and risk 107
Neisseria gonorrhoeae 106
Neisseria meningitidis 98
North America 10
    cholera 28
    food poisoning 70, 72, 82
    hepatitis B 34
    Lyme disease 34–5, 96
    meningococcal disease 98
    pertussis 36
    plague 97
    poisonous spiders 122
    poliomyelitis 81
    rabies 101, 102
    relapsing fever 96
    scorpions 122
    spotted fever 94
    typhus 82

onchocerciasis 9, 11, 88–9, 126, 127, 131–43
otitis media and risk 19

parasitaemia, malarial 42, 43, 54
parasites and travellers' diarrhoea 64–5, 68–71
    returned travellers 126–7

see also Giardia; and others by name
penicillins 99, 127
pertussis vaccine, 30, 36
plague 10, 11, 12, 97, 125
    endemic areas 131–43
Plasmodium falciparum 11, 15, 41, 42, 43, 44, 45, 46, 49, 52, 53, 54; see also malaria
Plasmodium malariae 41, 42
Plasmodium ovale 41, 42, 43, 44, 53, 54
Plasmodium vivax 41, 42, 43, 44, 52, 53, 54
pneumococcal disease
    vaccine 18, 32–3, 36–7
pneumothorax and risk 19
poliomyelitis 7, 10, 68, 80–1
    vaccine 16, 22, 23, 32–3, 37, 81, 131–43
pre-travel health assessment 5–8
pregnancy 6, 7, 14–15
    air travel 14
    food-borne illness 15
    high altitude 15
    malaria 14–15
    motion sickness 24
    vaccination 15, 31, 33
proguanil 15, 46
    see also malaria, chemoprophylaxis

quinine 52, 53
quinolones 67, 77, 79
    fluoroquinolones 80

rabies 7, 9, 10, 11, 12, 13, 101–6, 131–43
    returned travellers 125
    vaccine 16, 22, 32–3, 37, 103–6
rehydration 77, 79, 112, 113–14
relapsing fever 9, 96, 125
returned travellers 123–9
    brucellosis 125
    dengue 57, 125
    diarrhoea 123–5
    eosinophilia 126–7
    fever 125–6
    intestinal worms 90, 126–7

jaundice 127–8
leishmaniasis 89
malaria 125
plague 125
rabies 125
relapsing fever 125
schistosomiasis 85
typhus 125
yellow fever 125
rickettsial infections *see* spotted
fevers; typhus
river blindness *see* onchocerciasis
rotavirus 64, 68–9, 76

*Salmonella* 64, 65, 66–7
quinolone resistance 77
*Salmonella typhi* 79, 80
sanitation and hygiene, risks
where poor 38–9, 81, 107
schistosomiasis 9, 10, 12, 83–6,
124
endemic areas 131–43
praziquantel 71, 86
returned travellers 125, 126,
127, 128
sexually transmitted diseases *see*
gonorrhoea; *and others by
name or regions*
Shigella 64, 65, 66–7
vaccine 76
sleeping sickness *see* African
trypanosomiasis
snow blindness 112
South America 7, 10–11
angiostrongyliasis 81
Chagas' disease 86
cholera 79
food poisoning 70, 72, 82
malaria 42, 46
myiasis 90
onchocerciasis 89
plague 97
poisonous spiders 122
rabies 101, 102
relapsing fever 96
schistosomiasis 83
scorpions 122
spotted fever 94
tuberculosis 110
tungiasis 91
typhoid 38, 80

typhus 82
yellow fever 55–6
South-East Asia 11–12
angiostrongyliasis 81
cholera 79
food poisoning 68, 70
Japanese encephalitis 59,
60–1, 62–3
malaria 42, 45, 46
schistosomiasis 83
typhus 93
yellow fever 39, 55
spotted fevers 10, 94
sun-related illness 18, 111–12

tetanus
toxoid with diphtheria vaccine
29, 32, 110
vaccination 30–1, 38
tetracycline 67, 69, 79, 127
thoracic surgery and risk 19
tick-borne encephalitis 12, 62,
94, 95
vaccine 32–3, 38, 95, 131–43
tick-borne relapsing fever 96
*see also* relapsing fever
toxoplasmosis 15, 70–1
travel sickness 17; *see also* jet
lag; motion sickness
travellers' diarrhoea 5, 7, 9, 10,
11, 12, 13, 15, 17, 22, 64–78
aetiology 64–5
chemical poisoning 72–3
enteric pathogens 64–5, 66–7,
68–71
prevention 65–76
antimicrobial prophylaxis
73–6
prophylactic drugs 76
water disinfection 65, 72–3,
75
treatment 67, 69, 71, 73,
77–8, 79, 80
*Trypanosoma cruzi see* Chagas'
disease
trypanosomiasis 9, 10, 87–8, 125
endemic areas 131–43
*see also* African
trypanosomiasis; Chagas'
disease
tuberculosis 19, 109–10

returned travellers 125, 127,
129
vaccine 32–3, 38, 110
tungiasis 91
typhoid 7, 9, 10, 12, 79–80, 125
vaccine 16, 18, 22, 23, 32–3,
38–9, 80, 131–43
typhus 9, 12, 13
endemic areas 131–43
louse-borne (epidemic) 11, 92
murine (endemic) 92–3
returned travellers 125
scrub 11, 93–4

vaccines and vaccination 28–40
allergic reactions 28, 34, 38,
39, 40
availability 8, 49
children 17, 18
in HIV sufferers 22
in pregnancy 15, 16, 31, 33
oral 28
recommendations by country
131–43
*see also* cholera; hepatitis; *and
other indications and vaccines
by name*
varicella vaccine 18, 32–3, 39
venomous bites and stings 9, 10,
13, 121–2
*Vibrio cholerae* 66–7, 78, 79
viral encephalitides 11
viral haemorrhagic fevers 9,
endemic areas 131–43

water-borne diseases 8, 9, 15,
57, 64–82, 107, 109
*see also* travellers' diarrhoea;
*and others by name*
West Nile fever 9, 13, 62

yellow fever 9, 11, 55, 56, 57
returned travellers 125, 128
vaccine 16, 18, 22, 23, 32–3,
39–40, 55, 56–7, 131–43